HIV/AIDS-Test and Treat

AF530345

HIV/AIDS-Test and Treat

Editors

Atul Kakar DNB FRCP
Vice Chairman
Department of Internal Medicine
Member, GRIPMER Governing Body
Sir Ganga Ram Hospital
New Delhi, India

Samiran Nundy MA MChir FRCS FRCP
Emeritus Consultant
Department of Surgical Gastroenterology and
Liver Transplantation
Editor-in-Chief
Current Medicine Research and Practice
Adviser, GRIPMER
New Delhi, India

Foreword

BB Rewari

JAYPEE The Health Sciences Publisher
New Delhi | London | Panama

Jaypee Brothers Medical Publishers (P) Ltd

Headquarters
Jaypee Brothers Medical Publishers (P) Ltd.
4838/24, Ansari Road, Daryaganj
New Delhi 110 002, India
Phone: +91-11-43574357
Fax: +91-11-43574314
E-mail: jaypee@jaypeebrothers.com

Overseas Offices
JP Medical Ltd.
83, Victoria Street, London
SW1H 0HW (UK)
Phone: +44-20 3170 8910
Fax: +44(0)20 3008 6180
E-mail: info@jpmedpub.com

Jaypee-Highlights Medical Publishers Inc.
City of Knowledge, Bld. 235, Clayton
Panama City, Panama
Phone: +1 507-301-0496
Fax: +1 507-301-0499
E-mail: cservice@jphmedical.com

Jaypee Brothers Medical Publishers (P) Ltd.
17/1-B, Babar Road, Block-B, Shyamoli
Mohammadpur, Dhaka-1207
Bangladesh
Mobile: +08801912003485
E-mail: jaypeedhaka@gmail.com

Jaypee Brothers Medical Publishers (P) Ltd.
Bhotahity, Kathmandu, Nepal
Phone: +977-9741283608
E-mail: kathmandu@jaypeebrothers.com

Website: www.jaypeebrothers.com
Website: www.jaypeedigital.com

© 2018, Jaypee Brothers Medical Publishers

The views and opinions expressed in this book are solely those of the original contributor(s)/author(s) and do not necessarily represent those of editor(s) of the book.

All rights reserved. No part of this publication may be reproduced, stored or transmitted in any form or by any means, electronic, mechanical, photocopying, recording or otherwise, without the prior permission in writing of the publishers.

All brand names and product names used in this book are trade names, service marks, trademarks or registered trademarks of their respective owners. The publisher is not associated with any product or vendor mentioned in this book.

Medical knowledge and practice change constantly. This book is designed to provide accurate, authoritative information about the subject matter in question. However, readers are advised to check the most current information available on procedures included and check information from the manufacturer of each product to be administered, to verify the recommended dose, formula, method and duration of administration, adverse effects and contraindications. It is the responsibility of the practitioner to take all appropriate safety precautions. Neither the publisher nor the author(s)/editor(s) assume any liability for any injury and/or damage to persons or property arising from or related to use of material in this book.

This book is sold on the understanding that the publisher is not engaged in providing professional medical services. If such advice or services are required, the services of a competent medical professional should be sought.

Every effort has been made where necessary to contact holders of copyright to obtain permission to reproduce copyright material. If any have been inadvertently overlooked, the publisher will be pleased to make the necessary arrangements at the first opportunity. The **CD/DVD-ROM** (if any) provided in the sealed envelope with this book is complimentary and free of cost. **Not meant for sale**.

Inquiries for bulk sales may be solicited at: jaypee@jaypeebrothers.com

HIV/AIDS-Test and Treat

First Edition: **2018**

ISBN: 978-93-5270-387-6

Printed at: Samrat Offset Pvt. Ltd.

Contributors

Shrihari Anil Anikhindi

Divya Arora

Sairam B

Bobby Bhalotra

Vinant Bhargava

Kunal Chawla

Sanghamitra Datta

Veronique Dinand

Shilpa Garg

Lovy Gaur

Parul Goel

Atul Gogia

Shweta Mittal Gupta

Isra Halim

Atul Kakar

Dinesh Kaul

Jyoti Kotwal

Ashish Kumar

Kishan Majithiya

Chandra Mansukhani

Manishi Nautiyal

Rashmi Nigam

Jaswinder Kaur Oberoi

Reena Raveendran

Darshit Shah

Ajay Sharma

Akanksha Tandon

Roopal Verma

Chand Wattal

Foreword

HIV epidemic in India has witnessed an immense contribution from wide range of people ranging from skilled or partially-skilled dedicated field workers to the highly qualified technical professionals, clinicians and researchers. The epidemic has graduated over the period of last 30 years and has cruised through various phases that coincide with the interventions made at individual levels, community levels and organizational levels. Astonishing and tireless efforts have been invested so far in designing and implementing the health program interventions to deal with the epidemic through public health approach at national, regional and local levels by the government of India through state governments and various communities, organizations and individuals. The successful achievements of the public health prevention, control and treatment programs could never have been possible without the evidence generation by the researchers and technical inputs provided by the experienced clinicians that manage the illnesses and sufferings of the patients in clinics.

Evidence base of HIV medicine has evolved extremely rapidly in recent past globally, so much so that by the time the knowledge is accumulated in form of a chapter of a book, new evidence will await at the corner. A wealth of information is available on-line, in form of various guidelines and updates. Though crucial, often the on-line information baffles the end users, especially busy clinicians, to choose and apply the knowledge while managing the patients in the clinics. The clinicians deal with diversified situations in practice viz establishing the diagnosis of HIV, when to initiate the anti-retro viral treatment, what anti-retro viral drug combinations will be the most suitable for the patient, how to identify and manage the toxicities of the anti-retro viral drugs, prophylaxis and treatment for the opportunistic infections, management of coinfections, comorbidities and malignancies, prevention of transmission of HIV to others especially from mother to child and also after occupational exposure to infected materials, and palliative care or end of life care for those who need it. The widely available online information often seems in sufficient to aid a treating physician when managing an actual case in a clinic or hospital.

This book is a prudent attempt to match the requirements of those clinicians and practitioners who desire to know a snapshot of vast recent knowledge out there that can benefit them in managing HIV in their clinics or hospitals. Authors of each chapter of this book have displayed dazzling skills by spelling out often complicated and difficult concepts around HIV diagnosis and management in a way that will assist clinicians, practitioners, students, program managers, and others interested, while approaching the HIV infection. I hope the enthusiasm expressed by the team of authors is translated in practice. My best wishes are with the team.

I congratulate Dr Atul Kakar for this great book and the work he is doing for care and support to those infected and affected by HIV/AIDS.

BB Rewari MD FRCP FICP
AG Regional Advisor HIV and
Scientist—HIV/STI/Hepatitis
World Health Organization
Regional office for South-East Asia
Associate Professor
Department of Global Health
University of Washington
Seattle, Washington, USA

Preface

The Human Immunodeficiency Virus (HIV) is the etiological agent of the acquired immunodeficiency syndrome (AIDS). It belongs to the family of human retroviruses (retroviridae) and subfamily of Lentivirus and mainly reproduces in CD4+ T lymphocytes and monocytes/macrophages causing severe immunological impairment. With the advent of anti-retro viral therapy (ART) the mortality and morbidity with patients living with HIV/AIDS has decreased.

The HIV epidemic has seen three major clinical themes over the past few years. According to many authors, the first decade started in 1981, when we use to treat only the opportunistic infection, manage the crisis and HIV management was limited to palliation provided by primary healthcarers. However, from1991 onwards, with the availability of anti-retro viral therapy, the focus has become more on specialized medicine given by HIV specialists who have a better understanding of viral pathogenesis. From 2001 to 2011, we were in a chronic disease era for HIV management. This also included managing the effects of HIV on the kidney, liver, central nervous system, heart and bone.

Malignancies in people living with HIV/AIDS have also become another area of concern in the last few years. Even nearly two decades into the modern anti-retro viral (ARV) era, the risk of death continues to drop for people living with HIV. Many things resulted in a change in the lives of patients with HIV/AIDS.

These are enumerated below:

1. In the field of diagnosis, early analysis can be done. The 4th generation HIV test has added the P24 antigen which can permit the diagnosis even before antibodies against HIV are formed (seroconversion). The advantages of earlier diagnosis include decreasing the risk of transmission, immune protection and possible cure.
2. After so many years of the epidemic being amongst us we can talk of a cure in HIV. The word 'Cure' in the HIV setting has two categories. If the virus is totally eliminated it is called a sterilizing cure and if the virus continues to be present in the body but the viraemia does not require anti-retro viral therapy (ART) it is called a functional cure .
3. From the therapic point of view, all the major guidelines now suggest treatment should be given to all HIV patients irrespective of their CD4 cell counts. This test and treat approach improves the quality of life of HIV patients and also decreases the incidence of new infection. According to 2015 statistics, 0.05% of the world's population is currently newly infected with HIV every year. With an aim of getting all patients under the umbrella

of anti-retro viral therapy, this incidence should come down leading to a lower burden on physicians.

4. The other positive thing which has happened is doctor education. The care of HIV is now simpler and more and more physicians are getting involved as they are becoming familiar with the drug regimen and also with the complications of therapy. Because of this HIV management has become more like chronic care provided by primary care physicians.
5. We now have new and safer drugs to combat infection. Efavirenz 600 mg is an important front line drug included in many guidelines including those of the WHO. However, the drug was previously associated with many side effects including suicidal ideas. Recent trials have demonstrated that 400 mg of the drug is non-inferior to 600 mg over the period of 96 weeks to achieve virological clearance and with less side effects.
6. Another important drug which is used in management is Tenofovir disoproxil fumarate. Presently Tenofovir is also a front line drug in patients with HIV AIDS. Its use has been associated with renal toxicity, Fanconi syndrome like features and also osteopenia/osteoporosis. Tenofovir alpha phenamine is a novel type of pro drug which should be available in the Indian market soon. By switching over to the prodrug, the side effect profile becomes favorable with less bone and renal toxicity.
7. Another important drug which has minimal side effects is Dolutegravir. This drug is a second generation integrase inhibitor. It can be given to a naïve patient as the first line therapy and also to patients who are failing on many anti-retro viral third line/salvage therapies. It has got a good safety profile. The major side effects of the drug include mild nausea, headache and sleep disorder. However, the drug is new to India and we need to see the side effect profile and where it should be placed in the management algorithm.
8. Once a month therapy for HIV is an excellent innovation available in the form of an injection. It contains two drugs, Cabotegravir and Rilpivirine, which need to be administered in both buttocks. Studies have demonstrated that the viral load is well controlled upto 30 days with a single dose. This is one step forward toward controlling HIV infection by replacing the daily pill burden and also in patients with problems of compliance.
9. The last word has to be about the HIV vaccine which is the need of the hour. Following many unsuccessful attempts moderate efficacy has been demonstrated with RV144 and AIDS VAX B/E. However, we are still a long way from a commercially available vaccine.

Atul Kakar

Samiran Nundy

Acknowledgments

No book gets completed without help from its authors and we would especially like to thank our contributors for the efforts they made and the quality of their contributions to this book. We are also grateful for the encouragement and support given to us by Dr DS Rana, Chairman, Board of Management as well as Dr PS Gupta, Dr SP Byotra and Dr Kusum Verma, Dean GRIPMER (The Ganga Ram Institute for Postgraduate Medical Education and Research) who are always there behind us during all our educational activities.

Last but not least, we would like to thank Mr Parmanand Tiwari, Junior Executive, in our hospital who has helped us right from the beginning to the completion of this important publication.

Contents

Section 6: Special Problems

Section 7: Precautions

Section 8: Miscellaneous

SECTION 1

Basics

CHAPTER

1

Introduction

Roopal Verma, Atul Kakar

The human immunodeficiency virus (HIV) is a retrovirus infection which causes the acquired immunodeficiency syndrome (AIDS) (Fig. 1.1). It attacks the body's immune system; particularly destroying the CD4 T lymphocytes. This damage to immunity results in opportunistic infections and malignancies.

The first case of HIV was diagnosed in India in 1986 in a female sex worker (FSW) in Chennai. At that time, more than 20,000 cases had already been reported worldwide. Such a delayed detection of the first case in India was probably due to a lack of laboratory facilities and scientific knowledge about this disease in this country. The HIV prevalence in India among adults is now about 0.26% (2015 data); of whom 0.30% are males and 0.22% are females. Among the states, Manipur has the highest occurrence, followed by Mizoram, Nagaland, Andhra Pradesh and Telangana, Karnataka, Gujarat, and Goa. The total burden of people living with HIV (PLHIV) is approximately 21.17 lacs

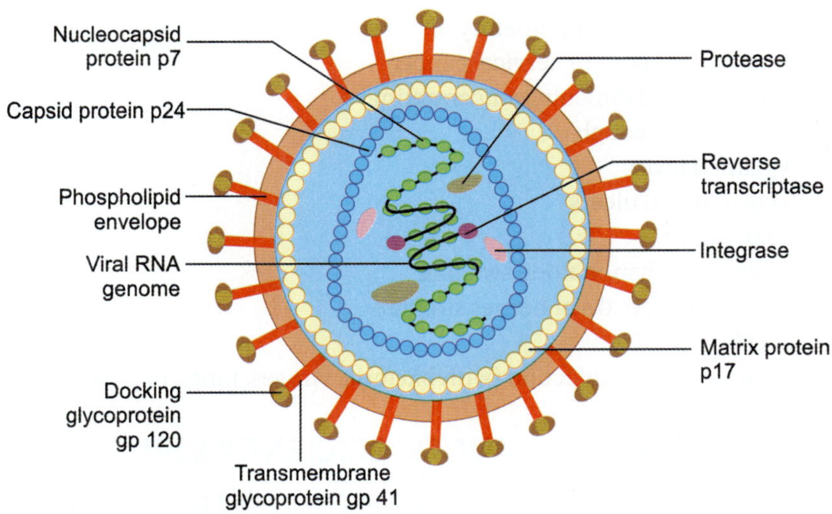

Fig. 1.1: Human immunodeficiency virus.

(in 2015); of which 6.54% are children and 40.5% are women. India is still facing an epidemic of HIV.

In 2015, the HIV prevalence in India was an estimated 0.26%. However, of the 2.1 million patients with HIV in India, only 43% are on antiretroviral therapy (ART). The Government of India's new goal is to stop HIV spreading by testing and treating all patients by 2030.

The HIV/AIDS can affect all sectors of the population, both rich and poor, children and the old, males and females, homosexuals and heterosexuals but its prevalence is greater in certain individuals who belong to the high-risk groups. These include FSWs, men who have sex with men (MSM), transgenders (TGs)/Hijras and injecting drug users (IDUs). The people who transfer infection from the high-risk to the low-risk group are known as the bridging population, which includes migrants and long distance truckers. In India, this infection follows, the so-called type 4 pattern where first the virus enters into the high-risk groups, then involves the bridging population and finally infects the general public.

WHEN TO SUSPECT HIV/AIDS?

The following are the clinical scenarios for suspecting HIV infection:

- All persons who are being evaluated or being treated for sexually transmitted diseases (STDs)
- Voluntary testing after high-risk sexual activity
- Recurrent infections in a person
- Unexplained weight loss
- Chronic diarrhea
- More than three vaginal infections in 1 year (not related to the use of antibiotics)
- Recurrent pelvic inflammatory disease (PID)
- Abnormal Pap test or cervical cancer
- Confusion and difficulty concentrating
- Persisting dry cough
- Explained fever
- Recurrent oral ulcers
- Night sweats
- Unexplained lymph node swelling
- Repeated outbreaks of herpes simplex
- Thrush
- An opportunistic infection (with bacteria, viruses, fungi, or protozoa).

ACUTE HUMAN IMMUNODEFICIENCY VIRUS

The HIV infection represents a spectrum of disease that can begin like a flu-like illness after viral exposure. This may be absent in some people and can be easily missed in many cases as the symptoms are very nonspecific. The symptoms of early HIV include headaches, fever, tiredness, swollen lymph nodes, sore throat, muscle and joint pains, mouth ulcers, genital ulcers, night sweats and diarrhea. Early HIV symptoms generally arise after 1–2 months of infection, although they can arrive as early as 2 weeks after exposure. Later Chapters in the book deal with how to test for HIV in the acute setting.

OPPORTUNISTIC INFECTIONS AND MALIGNANCIES

The HIV/AIDS patients are prone to many opportunistic infection and malignancies (Fig. 1.2). Many of these infections will be discussed in detail later; the opportunistic infections are related to CD4 cell counts of patient (Fig. 1.3). However, some of the clinical conditions are discussed in this chapter. These include—Toxoplasmosis and Penicilliosis.

Toxoplasmosis

This is caused by the intracellular protozoan *Toxoplasma gondii*. It usually manifests when cell-mediated immunity falls with the level of the CD4 cell count being less than 100/mm^3. Its mode of spread is through the consumption of undercooked meat and water contaminated with oocysts.

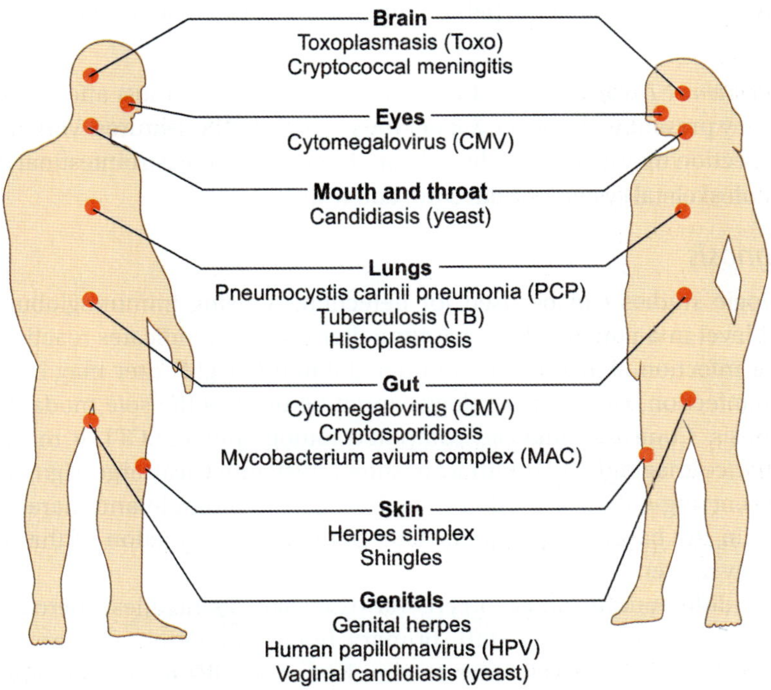

Fig. 1.2: Organ involvement in opportunistic infections.

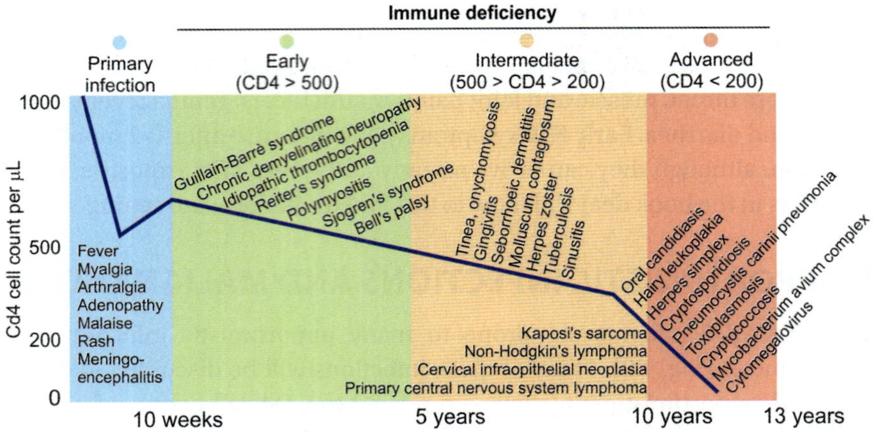

Fig. 1.3: Timing of opportunistic infection in relation with CD4 cell count.

Transplacental transfer has been reported in HIV-infected mothers resulting in congenital toxoplasmosis. The severity of the infection depends upon the trimester of pregnancy in which the mother has acquired the infection, being most severe if this has been in the first trimester.

Cerebral Toxoplasmosis: This is the most common and most fatal presentation of *Toxoplasma* infection. Usually the patient presents with altered mental status, headaches, fever, fits, unilateral limb weakness, difficulty in speech and vision, ataxia, cranial nerve palsies, and features of an increased intracranial pressure.

Extracerebral Toxoplasmosis: The eyes and lungs are the most affected sites, and may present without central nervous system (CNS) features. Very rarely, the infection may involve the liver, heart, bone marrow, gastrointestinal tract, musculoskeletal system, spinal cord, and testis.

Diagnosis

Serologic studies can be used for detection. A rising immunoglobulin G (IgG) level in a patient whose baseline titer is known indicates reactivation of the infection. A rise in the immunoglobulin G (IgM) titer may indicate acute infection. However, serology cannot be used as the sole modality for diagnosis. Contrast-enhanced computed tomography (CECT) or magnetic resonance imaging (MRI) brain scans show an asymmetrical target sign, which represent ring-enhancing lesions, which are usually multiple, and characteristically in the basal ganglia, brainstem, pituitary, and junction of the white and gray matter.

The differential diagnosis of cerebral toxoplasmosis includes tuberculoma, abscesses (fungal or bacterial), primary brain lymphoma, primary brain tumors, brain metastases, infarcts, arteriovenous (AV) malformations and demyelinating disease (Fig. 1.4).

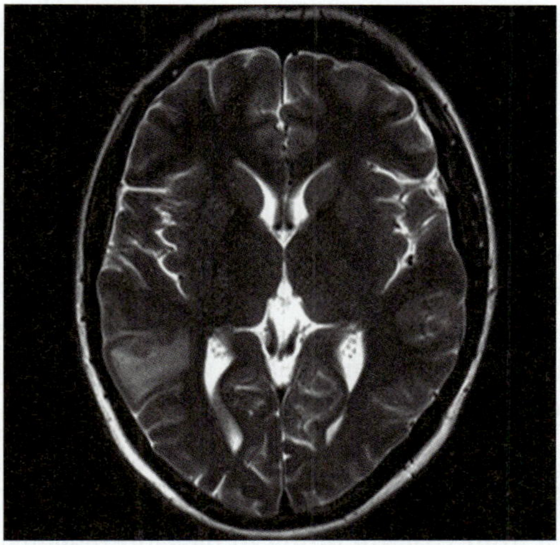

Fig. 1.4: MRI suggestive of space occupying lesion in brain.

Treatment

Primary prophylaxis should start with TMP-SMX double strength daily in *Toxoplasma* IgG-positive individuals with CD4 cell counts less than 100. The acute infection should be treated with pyrimethamine (200 mg PO once daily followed by weight-based therapy with pyrimethamine and sulfadiazine) and leucovorin. After completion of acute treatment, all patients should be initiated onto maintenance therapy.

Penicilliosis

This is due to a dimorphic fungus *Penicillium marneffei* which causes systemic infections in patients with HIV/AIDS who have CD4 cell counts less than 100 cells/mm^3. Southeast Asia is the endemic area for this fungus. In India, a new endemic zone has been recognized in Manipur.

The patient acquires the infection by inhalation of microconidia or from reactivation of a silent focus. Its clinical features are usually nonspecific (fever, anemia and weight loss). The patient usually presents with generalized skin lesions in the form of papules with central umbilication as seen in molluscum contagiosum, starting from the face and gradually spreading to involve the limbs and trunk. It may present with symptoms related to other organs such as the CNS, lymph nodes, liver, lung, intestine, and bone marrow. The definitive diagnosis is made by isolation or demonstration of the fungus in clinical specimens. An early diagnosis can be made by microscopic examination with Giemsa stain of a skin scraping, bone marrow or lymph node aspirate, which shows intracellular and extracellular yeast-like organisms with clear central septation.

To prevent the first episode of acute infection prophylaxis should be given in the form of itraconazole 200 mg once daily to the patient whose CD4 cell counts are less than 100/mm^3. Alternatively, fluconazole may be used (400 mg PO once weekly). Acute infection in severely ill patients should be managed with intravenous (IV) liposomal amphotericin B (3–5 mg/kg/day for 2 weeks) followed by itraconazole (200 mg PO BID for 10 weeks). Milder infections can be treated with itraconazole alone (200 mg PO BID for 8 weeks). The patient should then be continued on maintenance therapy with itraconazole (200 mg PO daily). Alternatively, an acute infection can be managed with voriconazole. ART should be started along with treatment of penicilliosis to improve the outcome.

HIV-RELATED MALIGNANCIES

Patients suffering from HIV are prone to develop malignancies. There are types which are—AIDS-defining cancers (ADCs) and non-AIDS-defining cancers (NADCs). With the introduction of highly active antiretroviral therapy (HAART), the cases of ADCs have reduced significantly.

AIDS-defining cancers: They are Kaposi's sarcoma (KS), primary CNS lymphoma, non-Hodgkin's lymphoma (NHL), and cervical cancer. ADCs reflect the point at which HIV infection has progressed to AIDS. KS is a low-grade soft tissue tumor of vascular origin, and it is associated with human herpesvirus 8 (HHV-8) infection. Manifestations of KS range from asymptomatic skin lesions to symptom producing visceral (lung and intestine) or oral lesions. NHL is a malignancy of the lymphoid tissue. In HIV/AIDS patients, the important risk factors for the development of NHL are a low CD4 count, high viral load, increasing age, and male gender. The World Health Organization (WHO) has divided AIDS-related lymphomas (ARLs) into three groups:

1. Those also found in immunocompetent patients like Burkitt's or diffuse large B-cell lymphoma.
2. Those found more specifically in HIV-infected patients like primary effusion lymphoma, and plasmablastic lymphoma.
3. Those also occurring in other immunodeficiency states such as post-transplant lymphoproliferative disorders.

Certain viruses also play important roles in NHL such as Epstein-Barr virus (EBV) and HHV-8. The incidence of invasive cervical carcinoma is increased in HIV/AIDS-infected females mainly due to infection by the human papillomavirus (HPV).

Non-AIDS-defining cancers: The incidence of NADCs has increased greater than three fold in the last 10 years. This increase is due to the longer survivals in the combination ART (cART) era and due to the direct effect of HIV itself.

All of these malignancies may found in HIV patients but their occurrence does not imply progression to AIDS. These NADCs are bronchogenic carcinoma, colorectal carcinoma, anal carcinoma, prostate carcinoma, testicular carcinoma, melanomas, Hodgkin's disease and cutaneous malignancies.

CONCLUSION

- HIV/AIDS is a infection usually spreads by sexual contact (hetrosexual).
- Patients with HIV/AIDS are more prone for opportunistic infection caused by bacterial, fungi and parasites.
- Patients with AIDS have more risk of cancers like Kaposi's sarcoma, Burkitt's lymphoma, primary CNS lymphoma and cervical cancer.

SUGGESTED READING

1. Buchacz K, Baker RK, Palella FJ, Jr., et al. AIDS-defining opportunistic illnesses in US patients, 1994-2007: a cohort study. AIDS. 2010;24(10):1549-59.
2. http://naco.gov.in/about-us/policies-guidelines. Opportunistic Infections and Their Management National AIDS Control Organisation. Lasted accessed on 02.01.2018.
3. https://aidsinfo.nih.gov/guidelines. Guidelines for Prevention and Treatment of Opportunistic Infections in HIV-Infected Adults and Adolescents. Last accessed on 27.12.2017
4. Jones JL, Kruszon-Moran D, Sanders-Lewis K, et al. Toxoplasma gondii infection in the United States, 1994-2004, decline from the prior decade. Am J Trop Med Hyg. 2007;77(3):405-10.
5. Patel PK, Erlandsen JE, Kirkpatrick WR, et al. The changing epidemiology of oropharyngeal candidiasis in patients with HIV/AIDS in the era of antiretroviral therapy. AIDS Res Treat. doi: 10.1155/2012/262471.
6. Rottingen JA, Cameron DW, Garnett GP. A systematic review of the epidemiologic interactions between classic sexually transmitted diseases and HIV: how much really is known? Sex Transm Dis. 2001;28(10):579-97.
7. Wheat LJ, Connolly-Stringfield PA, Baker RL, et al. Disseminated histoplasmosis in the acquired immune deficiency syndrome: clinical findings, diagnosis and treatment, and review of the literature. Medicine (Baltimore). 1990;69(6):361-74.
8. World Health Organization. Global Tuberculosis Report. Geneva: World Health Organization; 2015. Available at http://apps.who.int/iris/bitstream/10665/191102/1/9789241565059_eng.pdf.

CHAPTER 2

Laboratory Diagnosis of HIV/AIDS Infection

Sanghamitra Datta

INTRODUCTION

The acquired immunodeficiency syndrome (AIDS) was first documented amongst homosexual men in America in 1981. A few years later, its causative organism—the human immunodeficiency virus (HIV) was discovered. Today sub-Saharan Africa and parts of Asia are the worst affected areas. According to the National AIDS Control Organization (NACO), the HIV/AIDS epidemic in India started in the year 1986–1987 with the first positive HIV case reported from Chennai, and the first diagnosed AIDS case was from Mumbai. According to the World Health Organization (WHO) data, India with 2.4 million people affected by HIV ranks second in the world only after sub-Saharan Africa.

DETECTION OF HIV

Laboratory tests detect and confirm the HIV status of a person. The choice and sensitivity of laboratory tests depends on the stage of infection. The time of detection of the viral components like the ribonucleic acid (RNA)/complementary deoxyribonucleic acid (cDNA)/p24 antigen and HIV antibodies are variable. Choosing the right laboratory test ensures a correct and confirmed diagnosis.

HIV Detection Window

The time of detection of each of the viral components following infection are 7–10 days after infection for HIV viral RNA, 10–20 days after infection for HIV p24 antigen and 20–30 days for HIV antibody. Figure 2.1 gives a clear picture of the serocon version window.

Stages of HIV

Following infection with the virus the patient goes through an eclipse phase. In this phase, all the viral components are undetectable and all the tests are negative.

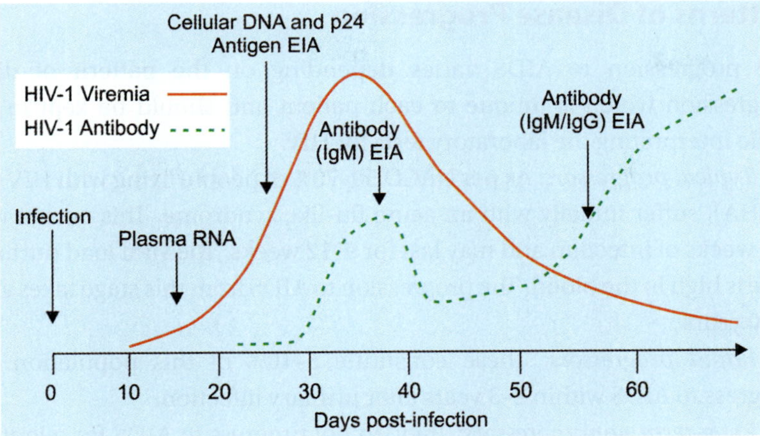

Fig. 2.1: Host response to HIV.

The eclipse stage is followed by three stages of infection: (1) acute stage, (2) chronic asymptomatic stage, (3) AIDS.

Acute HIV Infection Stage

This stage follows the eclipse stage. It is a transient nonspecific clinical syndrome associated with high viral replication which becomes detectable around 10 days after HIV infection. The acute stage usually lasts for a period of 3 weeks to a maximum of 6 weeks. The HIV antibody test is negative at this stage. The infectivity is high due to the absence of neutralizing antibodies and the viral burden is also high in the plasma and genital secretions. As the majority of people at this stage have common symptoms similar to any viral glandular fever, the diagnosis is missed in 80% of them. According to some authors half of HIV transmissions are by those who have a recent history of seroconversion which is less than 6 months. Hence, early detection of HIV infection is important in decreasing its spread.

Chronic Asymptomatic Phase

In this phase, antibodies are present and enzyme-linked immunosorbent assay (ELISA) for HIV antibody is positive. The presence of antibody down regulates viremia. Most of the HIV infections are diagnosed at this stage during screening which lasts for almost 10 years.

Acquired Immunodeficiency Syndrome

This stage lasts for 3 years or even less. The CD4 cells are destroyed steadily by the virus and the count falls below 200 cells/mm^3. The plasma viral counts increases and due to immune paralysis the antibody response gradually goes down and become negative. P24 antigen and the viral load test are positive.

Patterns of Disease Progression

The progression to AIDS varies depending on the pattern of disease progression which is unique to each patient and should be kept in mind while interpreting the laboratory tests for HIV.

Typical progressors: As per NACO 50–70% of people living with HIV/AIDS (PLHA), suffer initially with an acute flu-like syndrome. This occurs within 3–6 weeks of infection and may last for 9–12 weeks. The viral load during this time is high in the blood. The progression to AIDS from this stage takes almost 8–10 years.

Rapid progressors: These constitute 5–10% of this population. They progress to AIDS within 2–3 years after primary infection.

Long-term nonprogressors: They do not progress to AIDS for a long time even without treatment. Their viral counts remain less than 5,000 HIV RNA copies/mL. About 5% of patients fall into this category. Inherited mutations of the CCR5 receptor of T cell lymphocytes keep the virus under check.

Elite controllers: They are natural controllers of the disease and are a subset of long-term nonprogressors (LTNPs). Despite being infected, they can successfully suppress the virus to levels below 50 copies/mL for many years without therapy.

WHO and NACO have laid down the objectives of HIV testing. These are:

- To ensure safety of blood and blood products: there should be mandatory testing of all donated blood units and blood products
- To screening organ, sperm and tissue donors
- HIV screening in clinically suspected cases
- Antenatal care (ANC)
- Patients with tuberculosis, sexually transmitted diseases, high-risk behavior, hepatitis B and hepatitis C coinfection
- Epidemiological surveillance
- Research.

LABORATORY DIAGNOSIS

The HIV infection can be diagnosed by testing any of the following:

- Antibodies to HIV
- P24 HIV antigen
- HIV nucleic acid (RNA/DNA).

All antibody-based tests are divided into two: (1) screening test and (2) supplemental test.

1. Screening assays:
   - Enzyme-linked immunosorbent assay
   - Rapid screening tests.

2. Supplemental assays:
   - Immunofluorescence assay (IFA)
   - Western blot assay
   - Line immunoassay (LIA)
   - Radioimmunoprecipitation assay (RIPA).

Other assays apart from screening and supplemental tests are:

1. Molecular assays
2. P24 antigen detection
3. Culture.

Alternate tests and specimens are:

1. Oral fluid/saliva
2. Urine.

Antibody-based Tests

Screening Assays

Enzyme-linked immunosorbent assay: This is a screening test for HIV detection. The HIV antibody can be detected within 6–12 weeks in most cases. The fourth-generation ELISA test which is used today has the ability to detect both p24 antigen and HIV antibody and reduces the window period to 15–20 days.

According to the national HIV testing policy by NACO, two enzyme immunoassays (EIAs) using different principles together with a rapid assay are required to diagnose an HIV infection in a clinical setting.

Factors uniformly known to affect serological test results and are not recommended for testing as per NACO are:

- Hemolyzed samples
- Lipemic samples
- Repeated freezing and thawing
- Improperly stored, expired and deteriorated reagents.

Known common causes false-positive results are:

- Autoimmune diseases
- Alcoholic hepatitis
- Leprosy
- Multiple pregnancies
- Multiple transfusions.

Causes of false-negative results are:

- Window period
- Immunosuppressive therapy
- Immunological dysfunction (B cell disease)
- Last stage of the disease: immune collapse.

Rapid HIV tests: These are visual point-of-care tests and can yield results in less than 30 minutes. Though manufacturers have reported their sensitivities as 99.3–100% and specificity as 99.7–99.9%, many studies have reported lower sensitivities and specificities.

Rapid tests recommended by NACO:

- Immunoconcentration/dot blot immunoassay (vertical flow), immunochromatographic (lateral flow)
- Particle agglutination (e.g. gelatin or latex test)
- Fluorimetric microparticle technology.

Advantage: Differentiates HIV-1 and HIV-2.

Disadvantage: Subjective interpretation is one of its major disadvantages.

The NACO has recommended that ELISA kits and rapid kits used must have high sensitivity and specificity (>99.5%, >98% respectively).

Supplemental Tests

Western blot assay: This is a specific test and is the most commonly used of all the supplemental assays. It has a lower positive predictive value when performed alone. HIV-1 Western blot and HIV-1 IFA were previously recommended to make a laboratory diagnosis of HIV-1 infection. These assays are not a part of the recommended algorithm as per the NACO guidelines. The various HIV-specific recombinant or synthetic antigens are electrophoresed onto nitrocellulose paper. Western blot detects the presence of antibodies against specific HIV proteins: Envelope (ENV; gp120, gp160 and gp41), GAG (p55, p24 and p17), POL (p66, p51 and p31). They are seen as bands on the test strip. The criterion for a positive Western blot is different for WHO and the Centers for Disease Control (CDC) in the United States. Table 2.1 gives the details of these.

The WHO criterion is most commonly used.

Interpretation:

Negative: No bands

Positive: Bands as given in Table 2.1.

Intermediate: Bands present that do not satisfy the criteria.

Western blot assay is only used now in case of an equivocal or discordant test (Figs. 2.2 and 2.3).

Line immunoassay: In this assay, the use of "artificial" antigens decreases the presence of contaminating substances derived from cell culture making it more specific.

Immunofluorescence assay and RIPA: IFA and RIPA are other supplemental methods which are not commonly used.

Table 2.1: Positive Western blot criteria.

Organization	***Criteria***
WHO	2 env with or without gag/pol
CDC	Any two p24, gp41, gp120/160

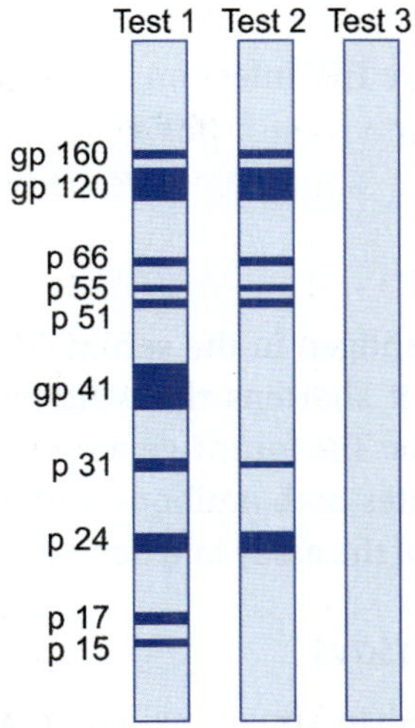

Fig. 2.2: Western blot. (Test 1) Control, as it shows all the proteins tested are present. Controls are crucial to make sure that the test is working correctly; (Test 2) Positive results shows there are antibodies for 7 of the HIV proteins; (Test 3) Negative result.

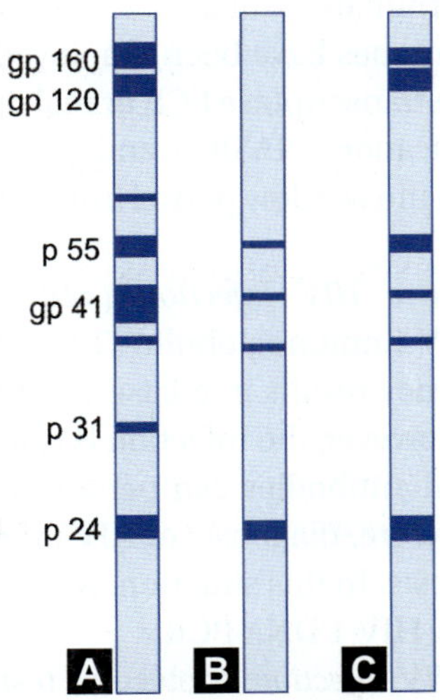

Figs. 2.3A to C: Western blot. (A) Control strip showing antibody responses to key HIV proteins; (B) Indeterminate response showing antibodies to p24; (C) Positive Western blot showing responses to at least three key proteins.

Other Assays

- HIV p24 antigen detection
- HIV DNA
- HIV RNA polymerase chain reaction (PCR)
- HIV culture.

Indications are as follows:
- Window period or acute HIV infection
- Indeterminate serology
- Neonatal infection.

P24 Antigen Detection

The test detects free p24 antigen in the serum. Though the detection of the p24 antigen is transient, it shortens the window period and can become positive as early as 2 weeks. The fourth-generation ELISA used nowadays as a screening test incorporates both antibody and p24 antigen detection thus increasing the sensitivity of the assay and decreasing the window period.

Molecular DNA/RNA Assays

These assays are indicated in situations where antibody detection assays cannot be relied upon. Molecular assays amplify both HIV RNA or proviral DNA. They are used for:
- Diagnosis of HIV in children less than 18 months old
- Diagnosis of acute HIV infection
- Resolution of indeterminate results.

Three different techniques have been employed to develop commercial kits. They are: (1) reverse transcriptase PCR or real time-PCR, (2) nucleic acid sequence-based amplification (NASBA) and (3) branched DNA (b-DNA) assay. These kits shorten the window period from infection to detection by 12 days.

Diagnosis of pediatric HIV infection (<18 months): Transplacental transfer of maternal HIV immunoglobulin G (IgG) from infected mothers to babies during pregnancy results in a false-reactive test in babies born to HIV-positive mothers. However, the infection is transmitted in less than 50% of such babies. Maternal antibodies can persist in an infant's blood for 18 months after birth. Therefore, diagnosis of HIV infection till this age cannot be done by serological tests. In this situation, NACO recommends the use of the test called qualitative HIV-1 DNA PCR.

Detection of acute HIV infection: Molecular tests are the tests of choice for diagnosing of infection during the "window period" also called acute HIV infection. A positive test confirms the diagnosis, but a negative test does not rule it out.

Resolution of indeterminate results: Specimens that are reactive on initial immunoassay and nonreactive or indeterminate on the antibody differentiation assay should undergo HIV-1 nucleic acid testing for resolution of the discordant result.

The RNA quantitative assays used these days have a low detection limit and are very sensitive. They are of great importance in monitoring the viral load especially in patients on antiretroviral therapy.

Alternate to Classical Tests

These tests have recently come to the fore. The samples are saliva and urine instead of blood that detect HIV antibodies in saliva and urine.

Advantages:

- Noninvasive methods of sample collection
- Appropriate for people who object to giving blood
- Safer to handle urine and saliva which contains less virus that is insufficient for transmission.

Oral fluid: Detects antibody and not virus in the saliva. OraSure is the only oral fluid test approved by the US Food and Drug Administration. Lower sensitivity than blood-based tests.

Urine: Detects HIV antibodies but not the virus in urine. Sensitivity is less than blood and oral fluid.

Disadvantage: There is no approved urine-based confirmatory assay necessitating collection of blood when results are reactive.

Social Aspects of HIV Testing

Legal aspects of HIV testing: NACO guidelines should be followed.

1. *Pre-test counseling*: The pre-test counseling is an integral part of HIV testing services.
2. *Confidentiality*: The confidentiality of HIV test results should be maintained for both positive and negative reports. The reports should be dispatched to the individual concerned or person authorized by the individual or to the clinician in a sealed envelope who requested the test. The records must be kept secure.
   Reports are not to be communicated via the electronic media.
3. *Mandatory testing*: Mandatory testing is usually not recommended in India. However, it can be done *only* for:
   - Screening of units of blood for donations
   - Blood products
   - Organs, tissues and semen donors to prevent the transmission of HIV to the recipient.

The national HIV testing policy as per NACO further reiterates the following:

- No person should be tested mandatorily for HIV
- No mandatory HIV testing should be imposed as a precondition for employment or for providing healthcare services and facilities
- Any HIV testing must be accompanied by pre-test and post-test counseling services and informed consent
- Confidentiality of the result should be maintained.

NATIONAL STRATEGIES AND ALGORITHM FOR HIV TESTING (NACO GUIDELINES)

In India, the objectives for HIV screening and its diagnosis are guided by NACO guidelines.

Three strategies for HIV diagnosis have been laid down by NACO for (1) blood/organ donation safety, (2) surveillance and (3) disease diagnosis.

The laboratory diagnosis is based on serial testing. This includes repeat testing on initially reactive samples (e.g. ELISA/ELFA).

The first, second, and third tests (A1, A2, and A3) are based on different principles and use different antigenic composition (e.g. different generations of ELISA, i.e. 3rd/4th generation).

Serial Testing Strategy

- Serial testing strategy refers to the use of one screening test followed by one or more other ELISA/Rapid (E/R) tests, depending on the results of the first.
- A nonreactive result from the initial screening test completes the testing, i.e. report is given out as HIV negative.
- If the initial test is reactive, it is followed by a single test (in a two-test algorithm), or two more tests (in a three-test algorithm) for resolution.

Screening Strategies

The following strategies have coined by NACO and should be followed.

Strategy 1 (Flowchart 2.1)

- Sample subjected to screening test
- If negative: Free of HIV
- If positive: Reactive unit is discarded and donor is not recalled
- Used for donation safety (blood, blood products, organ, tissues and sperm).

Flowchart 2.1: Strategy I.

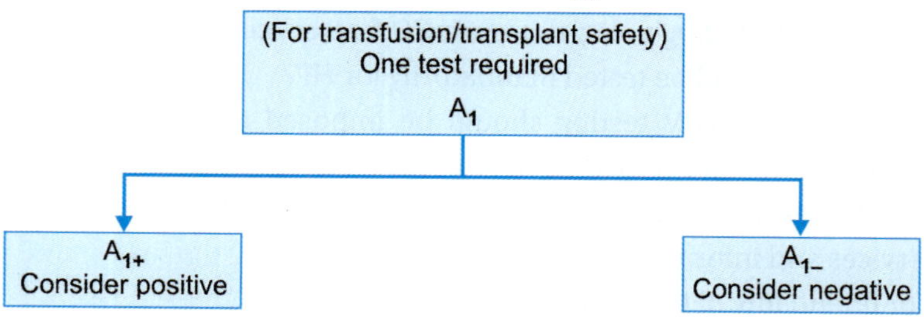

Strategy 2A (Flowchart 2.2)

- Used for surveillance A sample is negative if ELISA negative
- If reactive, second assay utilizing a different system from first.

Flowchart 2.2: Strategy 2A.

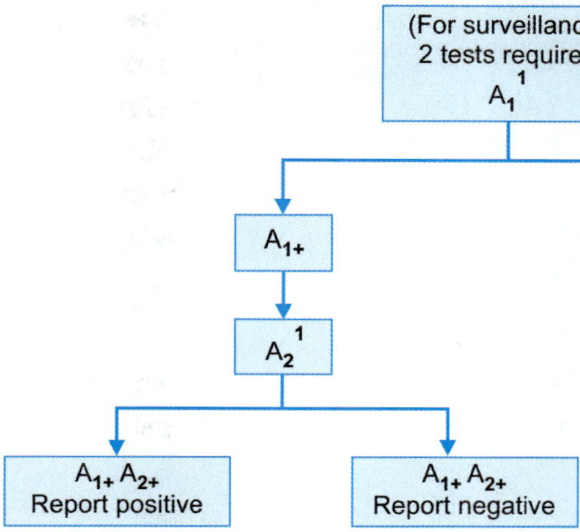

Strategy 2B (Flowchart 2.3)

- For diagnosis of individuals with AIDS-related disease and symptoms
- In case of indeterminate sample, repeat after 14 days.

Flowchart 2.3: Strategy 2B.

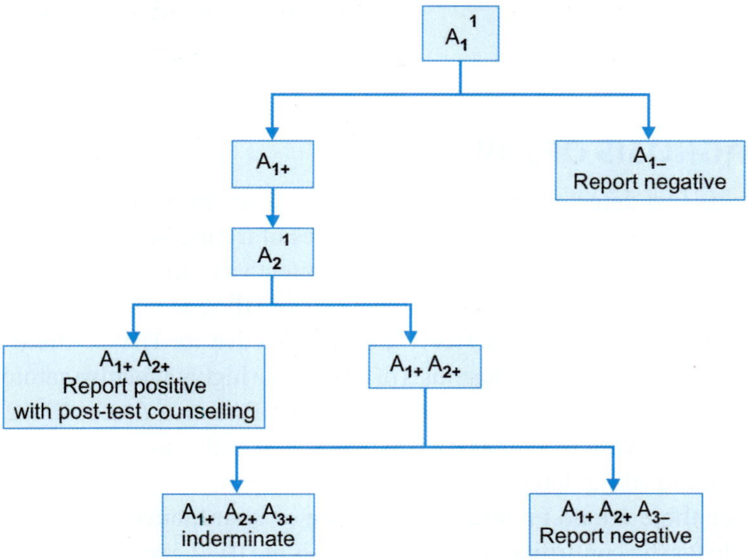

Strategy 3 (Flowchart 2.4)

- Same as strategy 2, with added confirmation of third reactive ELISA
- Used to diagnose HIV infection in asymptomatic individuals indulging in high-risk behavior.

Flowchart 2.4: Strategy 3.

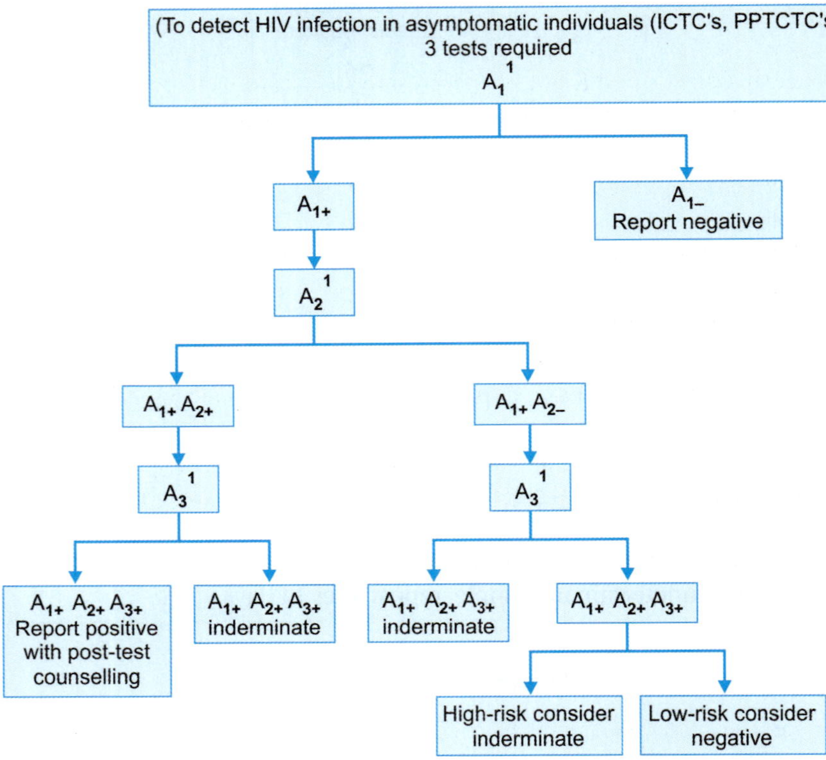

DIAGNOSIS OF HIV-2

HIV-2 was first detected from patients of AIDS living in West Africa. In India, it is detected sporadically. Though the modes of transmission are the same, it runs a much milder course in terms of infectivity. The progress to AIDS of HIV-2 is slower than HIV-1. The diagnosis of HIV-2 is important as some antiretroviral drugs used for HIV-1 are not effective for HIV-2. There is no exclusive algorithm for the diagnosis of HIV-2. The highly sensitive serological screening tests used these days for detecting HIV-1 also detect HIV-2. The supplemental Western blot assay is type specific and is available separately for HIV-1 and HIV-2 detection.

Since there are no molecular qualitative or quantitative licensed assays available for the confirmation of the diagnosis of HIV-2, Western blot is often used as a confirmatory test following a screening assay positive for HIV-2. Sometimes the detection of HIV-2 may be challenging in case of a repeated "indeterminate report" in a screening assay and a negative molecular test for HIV-1. In such cases, Western blot should be done to rule out HIV-2 infection as there are no recommended molecular assays for HIV-2 diagnosis in patients and molecular assays available for HIV-1 do not detect HIV-2.

CONCLUSION

- Early detection of HIV is of paramount importance to prevent further transmission of the disease as the infectivity is highest during the early stages.
- The strategies for diagnosis of HIV laid down by NACO should be strictly followed.
- Newer and improved screening assays have reduced the window period and hastened early detection. Legal aspects of HIV testing should be followed diligently.
- The pretest consent form should always accompany the sample to be tested, duly signed by both the doctor advising the test and the patient who is to be tested. In case of a minor, it should be signed by either the parent or guardian. The test results should be kept strictly confidential and positive results should be released with proper post-test counseling. In case of a high degree of suspicion, a negative result may not rule out infection and may be conveyed to the patient during counseling and the patient should be advised retesting after 4–6 weeks.

SUGGESTED READING

1. Alexander TS. Human Immunodeficiency virus diagnostic testing: 30-year of evolution. Clin Vacc Immunol. 2016;23(4):249-53.
2. Cornett JK, Kirn TJ. Laboratory diagnosis of HIV in adults: a review of current methods. CID. 2013;57:712-18.
3. National Guidelines for HIV Testing. NACO, July 2015.
4. National HIV Counselling & Testing Services (HCTS) Guidelines. NACO, December 2016.
5. Okulicz JF. Elite controllers and long term non progressions: models for HIV vaccine development. J AIDS Clinic Res. 2012;3(1):139-43.

CHAPTER 3

Human Immunodeficiency Virus Type 2 Infection

Akanksha Tandon, Atul Kakar

INTRODUCTION

West Africa is an endemic area for the human immunodeficiency virus type 2 (HIV2) infections where an average of 1–2 million people are HIV2 infected with the virus. HIV2 elsewhere usually occurs when there is a history of sexual contact or needles that are shared with infected persons of West African origin. In countries like France, Spain, Portugal, parts of India near Goa, the prevalence of HIV2 infection is high.

HIV-2 INFECTION

The general considerations for HIV2 infection are:

- Due to lower ribonucleic acid (RNA) levels, the infectivity of HIV2 is low.
- Similar to human immunodeficiency virus type, (HIV1) some of the HIV2 infected people develop an immunodeficient state and acquired immunodeficiency syndrome (AIDS) related complications but this develops slowly.
- There is generally a longer asymptomatic clinical stage in HIV2 infection along with lower viral loads in the serum. Compared to HIV1 seroconvertors viral loads are 28-fold lower in recent HIV2 seroconvertors.
- Mortality rates are lower compared to HIV1. However, HIV2 infected persons have a higher mortality once advanced immunodeficiency develops.
- Human immunodeficiency virus type 2 is associated with slower rates of CD4 decline.
- Concomitant HIV1 and HIV2 infection can also occur.
- As HIV2 is a less virulent virus than HIV1 there might be a possibility that HIV2 infection may protect against HIV1.
- Vertical transmission is much less common in HIV-2 infection.

People who are at risk for HIV2 infection; as per the CDC (Centers for Disease Control and Prevention) in the USA are:

- Sexual partners of a person from an HIV2 endemic country.
- Sexual partners of a person with already known HIV2 infection.

- People receiving either blood transfusions or an injection, which is nonsterile in an HIV2 endemic country.
- Children of women having HIV2 infection.

WHEN TO SUSPECT HIV2 INFECTION?

- People with HIV suspected illness but their HIV1 test result is not positive.
- Patients whose HIV-1 western blot suggests unusual indeterminate test band patterns of gag(p55,p24 or p17) plus pol(p66,p51 or p32) in the absence of env(gp160,gp120 or gp41).

DIAGNOSIS

- The confirmatory test for HIV2 infection is the western blot.
- Diagnostic tests for the detection of HIV2 infection as per the USFDA (Food and Drug Administration) use enzyme-linked immunosorbent assay (ELISA) and chemiluminescent immunoassays. These detect both HIV1 and HIV2 but cannot differentiate between the two.
- The multispot HIV1/HIV2 rapid test that works on the principle of immune-concentration is the only rapid antibody test that differentiates HIV2 infection.
- Multispot allows differentiation by incorporating peptide sequences which represent HIV1 and HIV2 infection.
- Confirmation with a supplemental HIV2 immunoblot test which is an antibody test should be done if the result is reactive for the initial serological antibody test for HIV2.
- There are no commercially available tests therefore in patients who are on treatment; it is difficult to monitor their RNA levels.

HOW TO MONITOR?

- CD4 cell count and clinical monitoring is recommended in all patients.
- For initiating antiretroviral therapy (ART) in HIV2 the optimal CD4 cell count threshold is unknown but it should be started before the onset of clinical progression.
- In HIV2 infected patients, the response of CD4 cell to therapy is lower than in HIV1 infection.
- Human immunodeficiency virus type 1 viral loads assay, which are commercially available do not reliably detect or quantify HIV2.
- Commercial viral load assays for HIV2 are not currently available.
- The virological response is difficult to monitor in the clinical setting.

THERAPY

- There have not been any clinical trials till date regarding when to initiate antiretroviral therapy (ART) or the choice of first line or second-line treatment for HIV2 infection.

- HIV2 appears resistant to NNRTIs and to enfuvirtide.
- HIV2 infection is nucleoside reverse transcriptase inhibitors (NRTIs) sensitive.
- Variable sensitivity has been reported to protease inhibitors (PIs) like lopinavir (LPV), saquinavir (SQV) and Darunavir (DRV). Therefore, due to their lack of ARV activity and increasing failure rates other protease inhibitors should be avoided.
- Integrase inhibitors, like raltegravir (RAL) and the CCR5 antagonist, maraviroc (MVC) are active against some HIV2 isolates.
- HIV2 infected patients on therapy commonly develop resistance associated viral mutations to PIs and NRTIs.
- For determining HIV2 coreceptor tropism no approved assays exist and in addition to CCR5 and CXCR4 HIV2 utilizes multiple minor coreceptors.
- Antiretroviral therapy naive patients with HIV2 or HIV1/dual infection should receive a regimen containing 2 NRTIs and a booster PI.
- For drug-resistant HIV2 therapy should be individualized and newer agents like RAL may be included.

CONCLUSION

- Human immunodeficiency virus type 2 infection is endemic for West Africa. Compared to HIV1 infection, it is less pathogenic but complications like immunodeficient states and AIDS-related complications may develop causing death.
- There is a need for RCTs to compare the treatment options for HIV2 infection. There are some laboratory testings for quantitative assay of HIV2 RNA levels in the plasma.
- The virus is resistant to NNRTIs and enfuvirtide but sensitive to some of the protease inhibitors like lopinavir, saquinavir, and darunavir. In addition to these, the integrase inhibitor raltegravir is also active against HIV2 infection.

SUGGESTED READING

1. Boyer PL, Sarafianos SG, Clark PK, et al. Why do HIV-1 and HIV-2 use different pathways to develop AZT resistance? PLoS Pathog. 2006;2:e10.
2. Brower ET, Bacha UM, Kawasaki Y, et al. Inhibition of HIV-2 protease by HIV-1 protease inhibitors in clinical use. Chem Biol Drug Des. 2008;71:298-305.
3. Damond F, Benard A, Balotta C, et al. An international collaboration to standardize HIV-2 viral load assays: results from the 2009 ACHI(E)V(2E) quality control study. J Clin Microbiol. 2011;49:3491-7.
4. Gottlieb GS, Eholié SP, Nkengasong J, et al. A call for randomized controlled trials of antiretroviral therapy for HIV-2 infection in West Africa. AIDS. 2008;22:2069.
5. Poveda E, Rodes B, Toro C, Soriano V. Are fusion inhibitors active against all HIV variants? AIDS Res Hum Retroviruses. 2004;20:347-8.
6. Visseaux B, Charpentier C, Hurtado-Nedelec M, et al. In vitro phenotypic susceptibility of HIV-2 clinical isolates to CCR5 inhibitors. Antimicrob Agents Chemother. 2012;56:137-9.

SECTION 2

Anti-retro Viral Drugs

CHAPTER

4

Anti-retro Viral Drugs

Manishi Nautiyal, Atul Kakar

INTRODUCTION

The current standard of care is a combination of at least three anti-retro viral (ARV) drugs from different groups, referred to as combination anti-retro viral therapy (cART) or highly active anti-retro viral therapy (HAART). The goal is to suppress human immunodeficiency virus (HIV) replication and reduce viremia so as to prolong life and restore immunity by slowing down the progression of the disease. Although with currently available ARV drugs, HIV cannot be eradicated but with treatment they improves the quality of life. The reason behind the inability to eradicate HIV infection from human body completely is the long half-life of the latently infected pool of CD4 cells established during the early stages of an acute infection.

Flowchart 4.1: Classification of anti-retro viral therapy.

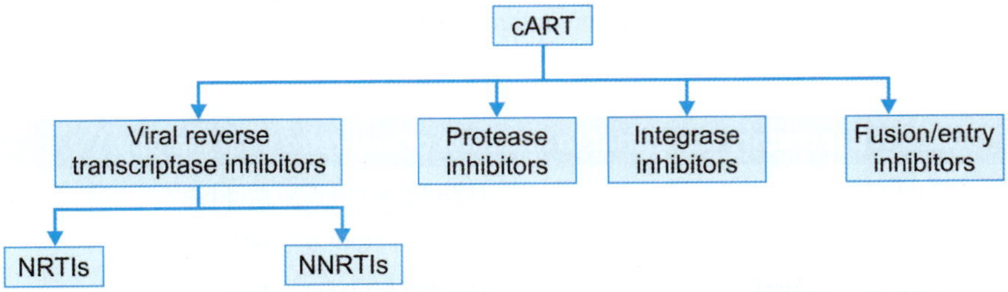

(cART: Combination anti-retro viral therapy; NRTIs: Nucleoside reverse transcriptase inhibitors; NNRTIs: Non-nucleoside reverse transcriptase inhibitors).

In India, 19 of the 26 ARV agents approved by the US Food and Drug Administration (FDA) are available. The selection of patients for initiating cART therapy is based on clinical, immunological and viral parameters. The adherence to therapy is of extreme importance and this should be ensured by appropriate counseling and education of patients about the disease. The rule is to initiate at least a three-drug combination therapy each drug from a different class. Monotherapy for HIV infection should not be used due to the relative ease of development of drug resistance. Nucleoside reverse transcriptase inhibitors (NRTIs) and nucleotide reverse transcriptase inhibitors (NtRTIs) are preferred for use according to the Department of Health and Human Services (DHHS). Flowchart 4.1 provides an overview of the classification of ARV drugs. Figure 4.1 depicts the site of action of ARV drugs.

Once the diagnosis of HIV is established, the following tests need to be performed to help determine the extent of the disease and to decide the best suited therapy for a particular patient as treatment needs to be individualized (Table 4.1).

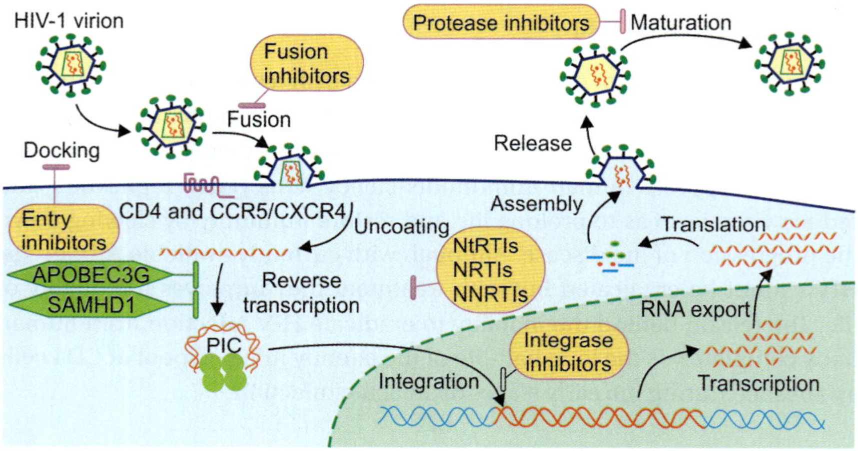

Fig. 4.1: Steps of the viral replication cycle pharmacologically targeted by combination anti-retro viral therapy.

Table 4.1: Laboratory tests prior to initiation of anti-retro viral therapy.

Complete hemogram	HBsAg, anti-HCV, anti-HAV
Biochemistry	PPD skin test or IGRA for TB
Lipid profile (fasting)	Record MMSE*
AST/ALT, total/direct bilirubin	Pap smear
Fasting blood glucose	HLA-B57:01 screening**
CD4+ T cell count	Toxoplasma antibody titer
Two separate plasma HIV RNA levels	RPR, VDRL test for syphilis
HIV-resistance testing	Pregnancy test†

*MMSE: Mini-Mental State Examination.

**HLA-B57:01 screening is done before initiating Abacavir (to avoid hypersensitivity reactions in patients positive for the HLA-B57:01 allele).

†Before initiating Efavirenz.

NUCLEOSIDE REVERSE TRANSCRIPTASE INHIBITORS

The NRTIs block enzyme reverse transcriptase in HIV. Table 4.2 gives drugs available as NRTI. All these agents can cause mitochondrial toxicity, i.e. lactic acidosis, peripheral neuropathy, hepatic steatosis and pancreatitis (Fig. 4.2). The manifestations of this may vary among the various drugs.

Table 4.2: Nucleoside reverse transcriptase inhibitor drugs.	
Zidovudine: AZT	Lamivudine: 3TC
Didanosine: DDI	Emtricitabine: FTC
Stavudine: D4T	Abacavir: ABC
Zalcitabine: DDC	

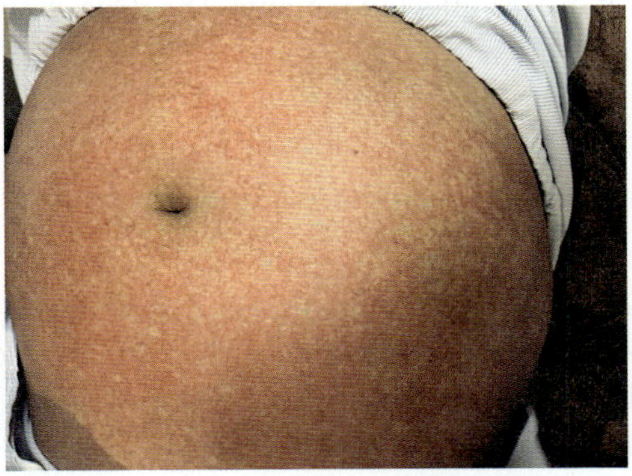

Fig. 4.2: Acute pancreatitis due to Zidovudine.

Zidovudine

Zidovudine (ZDV), also known as azidothymidine (AZT), is a thymidine analog, AZT being the first ART to be available. It has a good blood-brain barrier penetration. The dose is 300 mg twice daily or 200 mg thrice daily.

Side effects: Anemia, usually macrocytic and most patients on this medication have an elevated mean corpuscular volume (MCV). Anemia may develop after a month of use. Other side effects are granulocytopenia, hepatomegaly with steatosis. Elevation of transaminases, lactate dehydrogenase (LDH) and creatine phosphokinase (CPK) (myopathy) may occur. So when used initially monthly monitoring of the above parameters are indicated. It also results in nail pigmentation, nausea, headache, hyperglycemia, lipid abnormalities, lipoatrophy on long-term use and lactic acidosis (rare).

Caution: For renal failure (GFR—20 mL/min/1.73 m^2) or hemodialysis, reduce the dose to 300 mg once daily. For severe hepatic failure 100mg thrice daily is the recommended dose.

Emtricitabine

Emtricitabine (FTC) is a cytosine analog and the dose is 200 mg once daily. It is available alone as well as in combination with tenofovir or tenofovir and efavirenz (EFV). Resistance is associated with M184 mutation and K65R mutation in reverse transcriptase.

Side effects: Profile is mild like headache, nausea, diarrhea, skin rash.

Caution: Discontinuation of the drug results in flaring of hepatitis B in coinfected patients. FTC, lamivudine (3TC) and tenofovir disoproxil fumarate (TDF) also have activity against hepatitis B virus therefore when coinfected patients start or stop any of the three drugs, hepatitis flares due to the confounding issues of direct effects on hepatitis B virus, HIV, and immune reconstitution. That is why these drugs should never be used on their own for treating hepatitis B in HIV infected patients. The dose should be reduced in chronic kidney disease.

Lamivudine

This is cytosine analog and the dose is 150 mg twice daily or 300 mg once daily.

Side effects: Uncommon and include GI disturbances, headache and insomnia. Side effects are more common when used in combination with AZT and abacavir (ABC). It is usually well tolerated and is a part of a fixed drug combination.

Caution: It causes flare up of hepatitis-like FTC and resistance is associated with the M184V mutation. Resistance to 3TC occurs quickly. The dose should be reduced in patients with chronic kidney failure.

Abacavir

This has good CNS penetration and is well tolerated with very little mitochondrial toxicity. It is a guanosine analog and the dose is 300 mg twice daily.

Side effects: Hypersensitivity reactions (fever, skin rash, GI symptoms). Hypersensitivity occurs frequently in patients who are HLA-B57:01 positive. So prior screening for HLA-B57:01 is recommended. Rash (Fig. 4.3) and pruritus are seen in 3–8% patients within the first 6 weeks of use. Both of these are part of hypersensitivity reactions. In some patients, both may be absent and only fever can be the presentation. Rechallenging hypersensitivity can be fatal and is contraindicated. The risk of myocardial infarction has been reported due to a mechanism that is unclear. It is mainly metabolized in the liver.

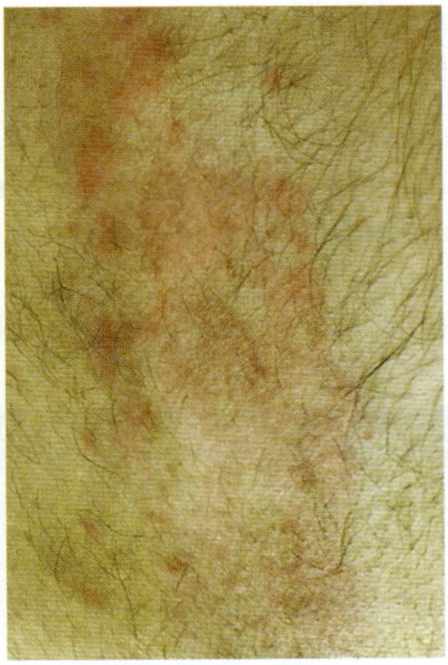

Fig. 4.3: Abacavir-induced rash.

Caution: In presence of renal failure (GFR < 20 mL/min/1.73 m^2), this drug should be avoided.

NUCLEOTIDE REVERSE TRANSCRIPTASE INHIBITORS

Tenofovir Disoproxil Fumarate

This is an adenosine monophosphate analog and the first nucleotide analog licensed for treating HIV. The dose of Tenofovir (TDF) 300 mg once daily.

Side effects: It is eliminated chiefly by kidneys and may cause renal impairment. Fanconi-like syndrome with hypophosphatemia may occur. TDF also causes osteomalacia. It is contraindicated in the presence of renal impairment. The creatinine clearance needs to be calculated and monitored in the first year of use.

Caution: Like FTC, 3TC, it also causes a flare up of hepatitis in coinfected patients. A prodrug analog of tenofovir currently in clinical trials is tenofovir-alafenamide fumarate—causes less renal toxicity. TDF is not recommended for patients at risk of kidney (creatinine clearance less than 60 mL/min) or bone disease (osteopenia/osteoporosis).

NON-NUCLEOSIDE REVERSE TRANSCRIPTASE INHIBITORS

Non-nucleoside reverse transcriptase inhibitors (NNRTIs)—Nevirapine (NVP), Efavirenz (EFV), Etravirine (ETR), Rilpivirine (RPV), Delavirdine—

inhibit HIV-1 reverse transcriptase. They are highly selective for HIV-1 and having no activity against HIV-2.

Side effects: Common to all these is a maculopapular rash developing within the first few weeks of therapy. Watch for the Stevens-Johnson syndrome (fever, mucosal involvement, painful desquamating lesions). These are hepatotoxic drugs.

Table 4.3 gives a list of commonly used drugs as NNRTIs.

Table 4.3: Non-nucleoside reverse transcriptase inhibitor drugs.	
Nevirapine: NVP	Efavirenz: EFV
Etravirine: ETR	Rilpivirine: RPV
Delavirdine: DLV	

Nevirapine

The dose is 200 mg once daily for 14 days then 200 mg twice daily.

Side effects: Fulminant hepatitis, hepatic necrosis and failure are reported with NVP (more common in women with high CD4 counts) (Figs. 4.4 and 4.5).

Caution: HIV/AIDS patients whose immunity is good (CD4 > 250 cells/mcL in women and > 400 cells/mcL in men) should avoid this drug and thus it is not recommended in postexposure prophylaxis. LFT is monitored biweekly for the first 2 months followed by once monthly. Stop this drug if the transaminases are elevated up to 3 times the normal levels. NVP has a favorable long-term profile especially on lipid levels. It has been used for a long time to prevent mother-to-child transmission.

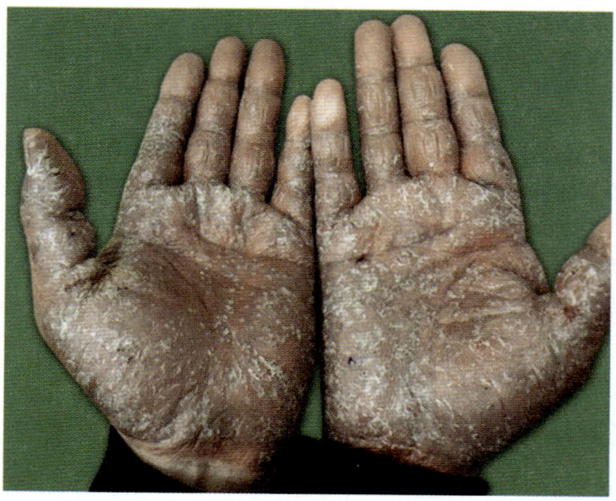

Fig. 4.4: Nevirapine-induced rash.

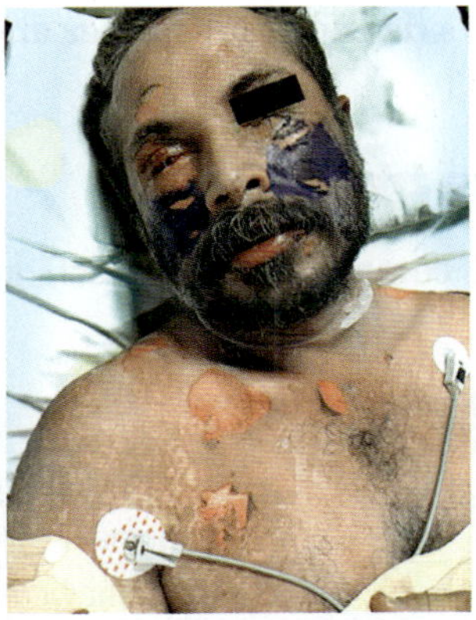

Fig. 4.5: Stevens-Johnson syndrome due to Nevirapine.

Efavirenz

This is the first line of therapy with a narrow therapeutic range and causes CNS toxicity.

The dose is 600 mg once daily at night time as it causes drowsiness and dizziness. It should be taken with fatty meals as the absorption is increased. In a recent trial dose of 400 mg EFV was noninferior to 600 mg.

Side effects: Efavirenz is neurotoxic, it causes confusion, dizziness, drowsiness, depression and vivid dreams. It also leads to dyslipidemia and is potentially teratogenic. The side effects usually wane over 1month's time.

Caution: It should be used with care in women of childbearing age and is contraindicated in pregnancy. Cross-resistance is not seen with ETR. It increases the risk of suicidal tendency (HR 2.6).

Rilpivirine

The dose is 25 mg once daily. It is less neurotoxic than EFV. This drug should not be used if the viral load is high (>100,000 copies/mL or CD4 is <200 cells/mm^3).

Caution: Proton pump inhibitors should not be given with RPV. RPV has fewer side effects than EFV making it an agent of choice.

Etravirine

It is a second generation NNRTI. Patients who have been exposed to first generation NNRTI can be shifted to these agents. The dose is 200 mg twice daily.

Caution: Patients with severe rash due to other NNRIs can be tried with this agent.

Side effects: The common side effects are nausea and rash. It is truly a second generation medication.

PROTEASE INHIBITORS

Table 4.4 gives a list of common drugs which are classified as protease inhibitors (PIs).

Table 4.4: Classification of protease inhibitors.	
Ritonavir: RTV	Indinavir: IDV
Atazanavir: ATV	Saquinavir: SQV
Darunavir: DRV	Amprenavir: APV
Lopinavir: LVP	Fosamprenavir: FPV
Tipranavir	Nelfinavir

HIV-1 PIs: Bind to viral protease and block the proteolytic cleavage of protein precursors that are necessary for the production of infectious viral particles.

Indinavir, Saquinavir and Ritonavir are rarely used first generation PIs because there are effective second generation PI. Indinavir causes nephrolithiasis (15%), UTI and indirect hyperbilirubinemia. Nelfinavir is the only PI for which Ritonavir boosting is not required.

Fosamprenavir is a prodrug of amprenavir. The major advantage over the former is the lower pill burden.

Side effects: Gastrointestinal symptoms and hyperlipidemia.

Ritonavir

The dose is 600 mg twice daily, it is also used in lower doses as a pharmacokinetic booster (100 mg or 200 mg once or twice daily).

Side effects: Nausea, diarrhea, abdominal pain, hyperlipidemia, hyperglycemia, fat redistribution and circumoral paresthesia. It inhibits cytochrome P450 3A4, thereby increasing plasma levels of the drugs metabolized by these pathways: Macrolides, R-warfarin, Ondansetron, Rifabutin/Rifampicin, most calcium channel blockers, Glucocorticoids, Statins, Sildenafil and some chemotherapeutic drugs used for treating Kaposi's sarcoma/lymphoma. It increases the activity of glucuronyl transferases thereby decreasing plasma levels of drugs metabolized by it: Acetaminophen, Digoxin, Diazepam, etc.

Lopinavir/Ritonavir Combination

This has more effective than Nelfinavir. The dose is 400 mg Lopinavir and 100 Ritonavir (2 tablets) twice daily with food.

Side effect: Diarrhea, lipid abnormalities. It is not the first-line therapy because of its side effect profile and high pill burden (Fig. 4.6).

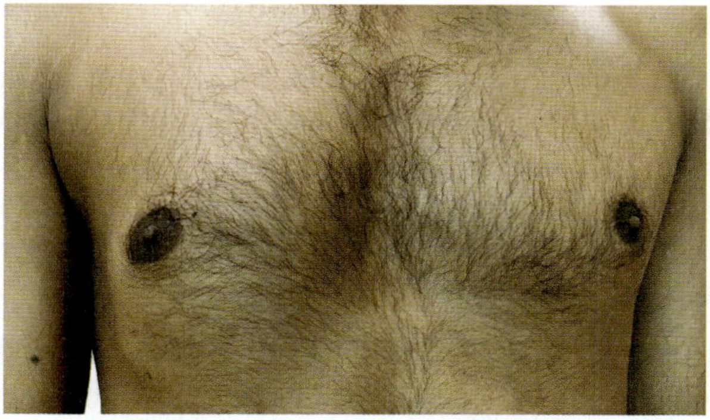

Fig. 4.6: Gynecomastia due to the combination of Ritonavir and Lopinavir.

Tipranavir

This is a nonpeptide PI. It is sensitive to some strains of HIV that are resistant to other PIs.

Side effects: Gastrointestinal mainly. Combination with Ritonavir causes damage. Cases of intracranial hemorrhage have been reported. It has a sulfa moiety and can thus cause allergies.

Atazinavir

The dose is 400 mg once daily or 300 mg with 100 mg Ritonavir in combination with FTC. The advantage over other PIs is that it causes less lipid abnormalities.

Side effects: Renal stones, elevates transaminases, causes hyperbilirubinemia (Fig. 4.7), hepatitis, PR prolongation on the ECG and GI side effects. It requires acidic pH for its absorption so a combination with a proton pump inhibitor is contraindicated. It also inhibits cytochrome P3A4 like Ritonavir causing elevated plasma concentrations of all the drugs metabolized by the enzyme.

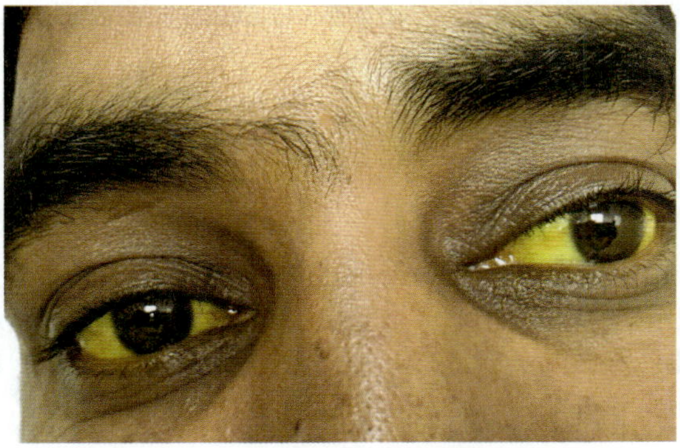

Fig. 4.7: Atazanavir-induced hyperbilirubinemia.

Darunavir

Darunavir (DRV) is a nonpeptide PI sulfa containing drug with a distinct chemical structure. This confers it with a high binding affinity and a slower dissociation rate, making it more 20 times potent than the rest of the PIs. It is active against multidrug resistant HIV isolates. The dose is 600 mg coadministered with 100 mg Ritonavir twice daily with food. It is in the list of recommended PIs.

Side effects: GI side effects are common to all PIs. Skin rashes may be related to its sulfonamide moiety. DRV causes hypertriglyceridemia, hypercholesterolemia, and raised levels of serum pancreatic amylase and lipase (>2 times upper normal limit).

Caution: It is contraindicated in patients on HMG CoA reductase inhibitors: simvastatin and lovastatin due to a risk of myopathy including rhabdomyolysis. Use the lowest possible dose of Atorvastatin, Rosuvastatin or Pravastatin with careful monitoring or consider other HMG CoA reductase inhibitors like Fluvastatin. It is contraindicated with Rifampin which is a potent CYP450 inducer and causes a significant decrease in DRV plasma concentrations.

INTEGRASE INHIBITORS

Integrase inhibitors prevent integration of HIV provirus into the host cell genome. This group is the safest and most potent of all ARV agents. All three agents show a more rapid decline in viral load compared to PI/r or NNRTI-based regimens. Table 4.5 lists drugs classified as PIs.

The three integrase inhibitors licensed are: (1) raltegravir, (2) elvitegravir, and (3) dolutegravir.

Table 4.5: Integrase inhibitors.
Raltegravir: RAL
Dolutegravir: DTG
Elvitegravir: EVG

Raltegravir

Raltegravir was the first approved HIV-1 integrase inhibitor (approved in 2007). The dose is 400 mg twice daily. It has good activity against HIV-2.

Side effect: Nausea, diarrhea, headache, rhabdomyolysis, CPK elevation, muscle weakness. Raltegravir is metabolized by glucuronidation, not metabolized by the liver; thus, the potential for drug-drug interactions is decreased. It has no abnormal effect on lipid metabolism.

Caution: It is an FDA pregnancy category C drug.

Elvitegravir

Approved in 2012, its dose is 1 tablet daily—always available in fixed dose combination with Tenofovir, FTC and Cobicistat: 85 mg or 150 mg formulation based on coadministered ARV agents.

Side effects: Diarrhea, nausea, headache and upper respiratory infections caution. It is not recommended if the creatinine clearance is less than 70 mL/min due to the Cobicistat component of a fixed dose tablet which inhibits tubular secretion of creatinine. Urine analysis should be done and proteinuria and glycosuria may be sign of tubulopathy. It should be taken with food.

Dolutegravir

Approved in 2013, the dose is 50 mg once daily for treatment naïve patients, 50 mg twice daily for treatment experienced patients or those on rifampin. Dolutegravir has demonstrated a response in patients who have earlier used other integrase inhibitors. Dolutegravir once-daily has a higher virologic efficacy compared with raltegravir twice-daily in a treatment-experienced, integrase inhibitor-naive population. It is commonly used in virological failure.

Side effects: Insomnia and headache.

Caution: Avoid coadministration of antacids or drugs containing calcium, magnesium, aluminum or iron because of chelation integrase inhibitors.

ENTRY INHIBITORS

Fusion inhibitors (FIs) and CCR5 coreceptor antagonists are two agents of entry inhibitors (Table 4.6).

Table 4.6: Entry inhibitors.
Enfuvirtide: ENF (fusion inhibitor)
Maraviroc: MVP (CCR5 antagonist)

Fusion and entry inhibitors: Interfere with binding of HIV to its receptor or coreceptor or interfere with fusion.

Enfuvirtide (T-20)

Prevents fusion of viral and host cell membranes (fusion inhibitor) by binding to HR1 region in the gp41 subunit present in the virus envelope of HIV-1, not active against HIV-2. It was licensed in the year 2003. The dose is 90 mg subcutaneously twice daily. Resistance is due to a change in its amino acid sequence at positions 36–45 of gp41. Its use is limited by the need for twice daily injections.

Side effects: It is well tolerated but is associated with injection site reactions (erythema, induration) and increased rate of bacterial pneumonia. Change of injection site is required.

Maraviroc

Maraviroc (MVP) is a CCR5 antagonist, licensed in 2007. In 2009, the license was extended to patients with R5 HIV-1 (treatment naïve). Therefore coreceptor tropism assay is mandatory before initiating this drug. The dose is 150–600 mg twice daily depending on concomitant drugs. If a patient is on a PI (CYP3A4 inhibitor), the dose is 150 mg twice daily. In patients on CYP3A4 inducers, the dose is 600 mg twice daily. In combination with NNRTIs, NRTIs, ENF, the dose is 300 mg twice daily.

Side effects: Upper respiratory infections (20%), arthritis and musculoskeletal symptoms (15%), rash (11%) and fever.

METABOLIC ISSUES AND COMPLICATIONS

- *Lipoatrophy*: This is the most common abnormality in HIV patients. The degree of lipoatrophy depends on the stage of disease. Those more immunosuppressed are at greatest risk. The underlying mechanism is mitochondrial toxicity induced by NRTI resulting in apoptosis of fat cells. Highest risk is with dideoxynucleosides—Stavudine, Didanosine, Zalcitabine, intermediate risk with AZT and lowest with FTC, 3TC, Tenofovir and ABC. Treatment consists of substituting Tenofovir/FTC for Stavudine/Didanosine, insulin sensitizing agents and plastic surgery. Figure 4.8 shows clinical features of mitochondrial toxicity.

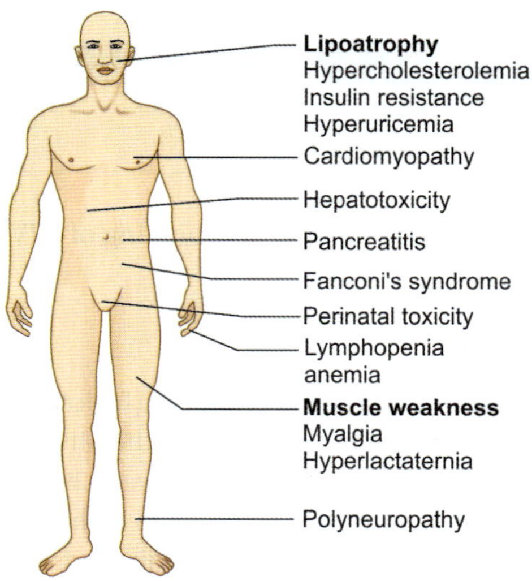

Fig. 4.8: Mitochondrial toxicity of anti-retro viral therapy.

- *Fat accumulation*: This mostly involves the neck (buffalo hump), upper body and intra-abdominal/visceral sites. Classically seen with PIs. No treatment modification has been shown to cause improvement. Exercise may reduce central fat accumulation. Rapidly effective technique is liposuction of neck fat which is necessary if its accumulation results in sleep apnea or neck pain. Figure 4.9 shows redistribution of fat due to lipodystrophy and Figure 4.10 shows grading of involving face.

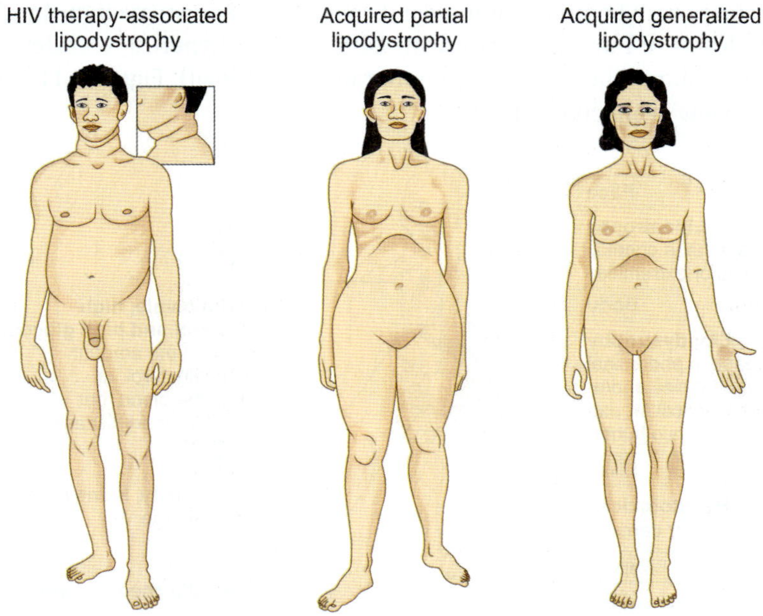

Fig. 4.9: Lipodystrophy grades.

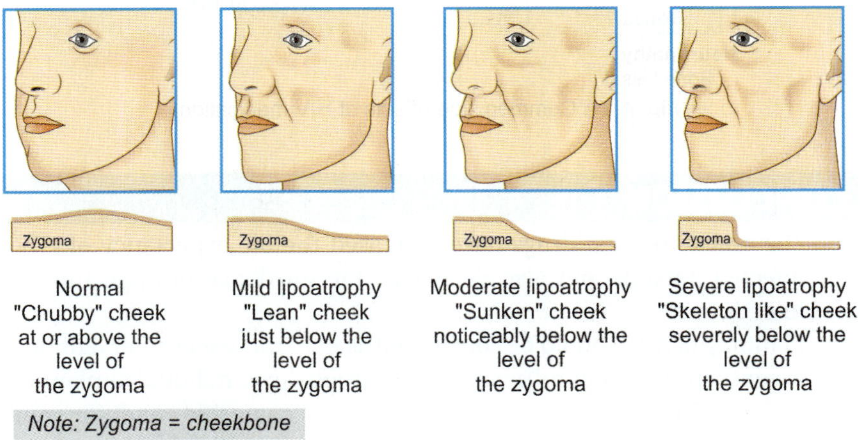

Fig. 4.10: Visual scale to grade HIV-related facial lipoatrophy.

- *Lipid abnormalities*: PIs are associated with hypertriglyceridemia and also hypercholesterolemia to a lesser extent. Other drugs known to induce lipid abnormalities are D4T, ZDV, ABC. EFV increases lipids, especially triglycerides, more than NVP, RAL and MVP. Elevation in LDL cholesterol will usually require statins. Most statins are metabolized by CYP3A4 except Fluvastatin, Rosuvastatin, Pravastatin. Use with PIs will result in elevated statin levels increasing the risk of statin related toxicity including rhabdomyolysis and hepatotoxicity. Not all statin—ART drug interactions are mediated through CYP3A4 as levels of rosuvastatin may increase with Lopinavir/Ritonavir through an unknown mechanism. Also the levels of Pravastatin rise with DRV. To treat hypertriglyceridemia, a fibrate should be tried first (fenofibrate/gemfibrozil). Figure 4.11 shows overview of effects of ART.

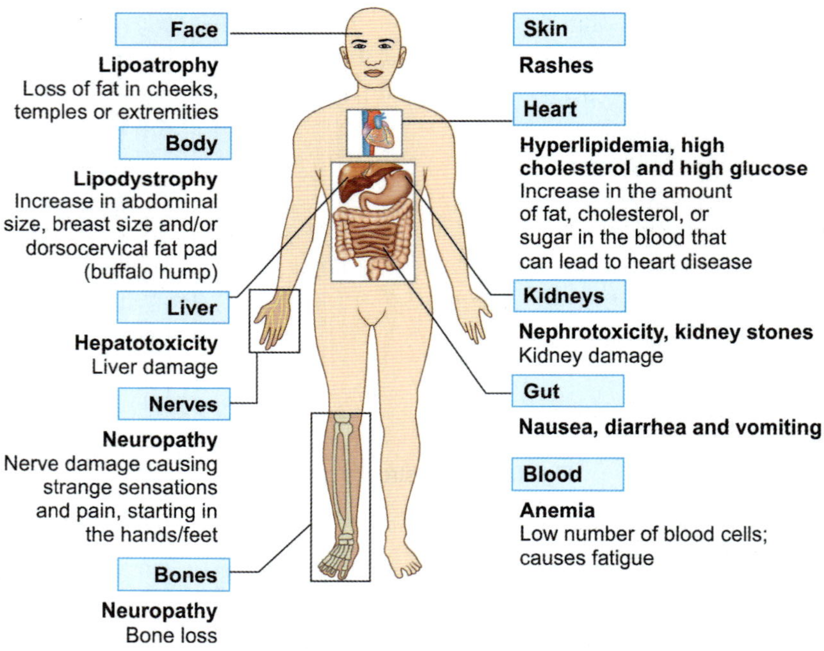

Fig. 4.11: Common side effects of HIV medication.

CONCLUSION

- The anti-retro viral drugs have increased the life expectancy of HIV-infected persons and also decreased the incidence of opportunistic infections.
- Planning of ART should be considered as nonemergency interventions, except in pregnancy and postexposure prophylaxis. It should be planned with consideration of its cost, the presence of comorbid conditions and its long term safety.

- For the seven agents which inhibit reverse transcriptase inhibitors (nucleoside/nucleotide), Stavudine and Didanosine are rarely used due to their side effect profiles. Didanosine causes pancreatitis and painful peripheral neuropathy whereas stavudine causes lactic acidosis, peripheral neuropathy and hepatitis.
- There are five agents which are non-NRTIs. They have also many advantages like a lower pill burden, few side effects and do not cause lipodystrophy. Patients with dyslipidemia due to PIs have improvement in their lipid profile. There is no benefit of using two NNRTIs at one time.
- There are ten PIs available. All these agents are metabolized by the cytochrome P450 system. Medicines such as Rifampicin which are known to induce P450 system should be avoided. All PIs (except Nelfinavir) should be used with Ritonavir. All PIs (except Atazanavir) have been associated with metabolic abnormalities such as elevated levels of serum cholesterol, triglyceride and insulin resistance.
- All patients on PIs should have annual lipid profile testing. There is a clinical interaction with statins. In general, the least interaction is with Pravastatin. Atorvastatin 10 mg orally or Rosuvastatin 5 mg/day may be used initially.
- Integrase inhibitors—slow HIV replication and are presently used for salvage therapy. Among entire inhibitors, ENF is injectable agent and Maraviroc works only against CCR tropic virus predominantly seen early in infection.

SUGGESTED READING

1. Arts EJ, Hazuda DJ. HIV-1 antiretroviral drug therapy. Cold Spring Harb Perspect Med. 2012;2:a007161.
2. Desai M, Iyer G, Dikshit RK. Antiretroviral drugs: critical issues and recent advances. Indian J Pharmacol. 2012;44:288-98.
3. Gunthord HF, Saag MS, Nenson A. et al. Antiretroviral drugs for treatment and prevention of HIV infection in Adult. 2016. Recommendation of the international Antiviral Society- USA Panel. JAMA 2016;316:191-210.
4. WHO. Consolidated guidelines on the use of antiretroviral drugs for treating and preventing HIV infection. Recommendations for a public health approach, 2nd edition; 2016.

CHAPTER 5

Anti-retro Viral Fixed Drug Combination

Dinesh Kaul

INTRODUCTION

Unusual cases of *Pneumocystis jirovecii (carinii)* pneumonia (PCP) were being reported in homosexual adults in 1981. This led to the discovery of acquired immunodeficiency syndrome and subsequently isolation of human immunodeficiency virus. This unique retroviral ribonucleic acid (RNA) virus was earlier classified as human T-cell lymphotropic virus-III. Within the span of a few years this infection had become a pandemic. Search for various anti-retro viral (ARV) agents led to the development of a thymidine analog, i.e. azidothymidine (Zidovudine) in 1986. Subsequently other nucleoside reverse transcriptase inhibitors like stavudine (d4T), Lamivudine (3TC) and Dideoxyinosine (ddI) were synthesized.

WHAT ARE FIXED DRUG COMBINATIONS?

Fixed drug combinations area formulation of medications where in two or more than two chemotherapeutic drugs have been added to have a better compliance without compromising the bioavailability and the efficacy of the newer formulation.

HISTORICAL ASPECTS

The first fixed drug combination approved by US Food and Drug Administration (FDA) in 1993 was Zidovudine and Lamivudine. With the introduction of Saquinavir in 1993, trials for a combination regimen of Zidovudine, Zalcitabine (DDC) and Saquinavir were carried out by Ann C Collier. However, this triple-drug ARV combination entailed taking a lot of pills by the patient. This high bill burden led to noncompliance issues and drug resistance.

Lot of ingenuity and pharmacokinetic (PK) studies led to the development of fixed drug combination in a single pill. Various pharmaceutical companies in India took the lead to develop such two- or three-drug formulation.

A combination of Zidovudine and Lamivudine was first developed by Cipla Ltd. and approved by the drug regulatory authority in India in the year 2000. Subsequently other drug manufacturers launched the same combination.

FIXED DRUG COMBINATIONS

Presently there are more than 10 fixed drug ARV formulations available in various countries which have been approved by their respective drug regulatory authorities.

Various formulations which are available in India include various nucleoside/nucleotide, non-nucleoside inhibitors. The most common drug combination used is Zidovudine and Lamivudine in most of the regimens. Stavudine was also used as a component of fixed drug combination along with lamivudine. However, various adverse effects of Stavudine like lactic acidosis, peripheral neuropathy, pancreatitis, lipodystrophy and metabolic problems have led to replacing this drug with newer and safer medications like Lamivudine or Emtricitabine. In the year 2000, the World Health Organization (WHO) advised stopping the use of Stavudine for routine use. However, it may be used in special circumstances when Zidovudine or Lamivudine cannot be used, especially when the hemoglobin level is less than 9.5 g/dL.

A list of various ARV medications available in India is given here:

1.	Zidovudine	+	Lamivudine	+	Nevirapine
2.	Zidovudine	+	Lamivudine	+	Efavirenz
3.	Abacavir	+	Lamivudine	+	Nevirapine
4.	Abacavir	+	Lamivudine	+	Efavirenz
5.	Tenofovir	+	Emtricitabine	+	Nevirapine
6.	Tenofovir	+	Emtricitabine	+	Efavirenz
7.	Tenofovir	+	Lamivudine	+	Nevirapine
8.	Tenofovir	+	Lamivudine	+	Efavirenz

Second-line regimens are given here:

1.	Zidovudine	+	Lamivudine	+	Atazanavir/Ritonavir
2.	Zidovudine	+	Lamivudine	+	Lopinavir/Ritonavir
3.	Tenofovir	+	Lamivudine	+	Atazanavir/Ritonavir
4.	Tenofovir	+	Lamivudine	+	Lopinavir/Ritonavir

These fixed drug combinations have led to better compliance and thus the morbidity and mortality due to the disease has also decreased. Newer ARV medications like Tenofovir, Emtricitabine and Efavirenz based combinations are used at present. These newer combinations are also approved in the pediatric population.

Initiatives taken by National AIDS Control Organization (NACO) in 2004 led to incorporation of the fixed drug ARV medications in the national HIV/AIDS control program for adults and children. The program has been implemented through various ARV centers across India. HIV-infected adults and children are given free care and ARV medication through this program. Initially the patients were given regimens of Stavudine, Lamivudine and Nevirapine or Efavirenz. Recently stavudine has been replaced by safer ARV agents like Lamivudine or Emtricitabine. Two regimens offered in the program use twice or once daily dosing. They include a combination pill of Emtricitabine, Tenofovir and Nevirapine or Emtricitabine, Tenofovir and Efavirenz.

PROTEASE INHIBITOR-BASED FIXED DRUG REGIMENS

Protease inhibitors are an integral part of anti-retro viral therapy (ART) regimens. They are advocated as first-line drugs in combination with nucleoside/nucleotide inhibitors. Various combinations with newer protease inhibitors are available in United States of America and Europe. These have been approved by various regulatory authorities. These include Rilpivirine (non-nucleoside reverse transcriptase inhibitor) + Tenofovir + Emtricitabine; Elvitegravir, Cobicistat, Tenofovir and Emtricitabine. Other combinations include Dolutegravir, Abacavir and Lamivudine.

Rilpivirine-based regimens have found to be noninferior to Efavirenz-based regimens in the context of viral suppression; however, the long-term failure rate and issues with possible drug resistance will be greater with this regimen.

Cobicistat (COBI) is a new PK inhibitor which acts as a boosting agent for few selected protease (Atazanavir, Darunavir) and integrase inhibitors (Elvitegravir). This is not used as a replacement agent for Ritonavir. It is only approved in adults and adolescents above 18 years of age. Various cobicistat-based fixed drug regimens are approved. This medication should be avoided in patients who are on tenofovir combinations and have renal insufficiency (creatinine clearance < 70 mL/min).

1. Emtricitabine 200 mg + Tenofovir 300 mg + Elvitegravir + Cobicistat 150 mg (Stribild)
2. Atazanavir 300 mg + Cobicistat 150 mg (Evotaz)
3. Darunavir 800 mg + Cobicistat 150 mg (Prezcobix)

Elvitegravir is a protease inhibitor. It is not to be used alone and should be used with a PK enhancer (boosting agent) like ritonavir or as a part of boosted protease inhibitor regimen or in combination with cobicistat. This is approved in adults and adolescents above 18 years of age. It has the advantage of once daily dosing.

The dosing schedules of Elvitegravir with various ARV agents are as the following:

1.	Elvitegravir 85 mg	+	Atazanavir 300 mg	+	Ritonavir100 mg
2.	Elvitegravir 85 mg	+	Lopinavir 400 mg	+	Ritonavir 100 mg
3.	Elvitegravir 150 mg	+	Darunavir 600 mg	+	Ritonavir 100 mg twice daily
4.	Elvitegravir 150 mg	+	Fosamprenavir 700 mg	+	Ritonavir 100 mg twice daily
5.	Elvitegravir 150 mg	+	Tipranavir 500 mg	+	Ritonavir 200 mg twice daily

A combination of Dolutegravir, Abacavir and Lamivudine is a simple regimen which can be used in adult population as a first-line medication, though the adverse effects due to Abacavir like rash, vomiting, fever and hypersensitivity reactions may pose a problem in certain individuals who are allergic to abacavir. Prior to initiation of abacavir, individuals may be tested for HLA-B*5701 allele. Individuals, who have this HLA haplotype, should not be given this medication.

FIXED DRUG COMBINATIONS FOR PRE-EXPOSURE AND POST-EXPOSURE PROPHYLAXIS

Various fixed drug combinations have been used for pre-exposure prophylaxis (PrEP) and post-exposure prophylaxis (PEP) to prevent HIV infection following a sexual or an occupational exposure. Ease of administration with a single or twice daily medication has made the prophylaxis easier reduced the pill burden and improved the drug compliance.

Recently a combination of Tenofovir and Emtricitabine *(Truvada®)* has been approved for the PrEP (sexual exposure), in discordant couples and in intravenous drug abusers as a single pill given once daily (2014). WHO has also endorsed this two-drug combination and guidelines on when to start ARV therapy as PrEP for HIV infection has been issued in September 2015.

The PrEP has been advocated only in emergency situations for unprotected sexual intercourse with an infected partner. This does not obviate the need for other protective measures or prevention of HIV infection like the use of barrier contraceptives. The prophylaxis is to be continued for 4 weeks.

In the setting of an occupational exposure to HIV infection, various fixed drug combinations have been recommended like Tenofovir, Lamivudine and Efavirenz in a single dose or twice daily with Lopinavir-Ritonavir combination instead of Efavirenz.

However, a new combination of *Tenofovir, Emtricitabine plus Raltegravir-Dolutegravir* has shown good results. The medication should be ideally initiated within 2 hours of a needle stick injury, blood splashes, mucosal exposure or any other exposure like biting by a patient, spitting or contact with blood-stained body fluids. The medication has to be taken by the healthcare worker for 28 days (4 weeks).

CONCLUSION

- A fixed drug combination lowers the pill burden for the patient and increases compliance.
- The drugs are formulated with an acceptable dose of each of active ingredient and are rational.
- It is a simple way to prescribe ART.
- Adherence, efficacy and cost are other positive efforts of fixed drug ART combinations.

SUGGESTED READING

1. Antiretroviral therapy guidelines for HIV-infected adults and adolescents. National AIDS Control Organization, Ministry of Family Welfare, Government of India, May 2013.
2. Baggaley R, Doherty M, Ball A, et al. The strategic use of antiretroviral agents to prevent HIV infection: a converging agenda. Clin Infect Dis. 2015;60(Suppl 3): S159-60.
3. CDC recommendation for postexposure prophylaxis (PEP) and non-postexposure prophylaxis. United States Public Health Service (USPHS) guidelines. 2015.
4. http://aidsinfo.nih.gov/contentfiles/lvguidelines/pediatricguidelines.pdf. Guidelines for the use of antiretroviral agents in pediatric HIV infection. (2017). Panel on antiretroviral therapy and medical management of HIV-infected children. Department of Health and Human Services. [Accessed October 2017].
5. Pazare AR. Evolution of anti-retroviral therapy: multiple pills to fixed drug combinations. JAPI. 2015;63:11-3.
6. US Public Health Services. Pre-exposure prophylaxis for the prevention of HIV infection in United States; 2014.

SECTION 3

Treatment

CHAPTER 6

When to Initiate Anti-retro Viral Therapy?

Atul Gogia, Atul Kakar

INTRODUCTION

Management of human immunodeficiency virus (HIV) infection over the past few years has witnessed several significant developments. The treatment involves the use of a combination of anti-retro viral drugs and the early initiation of these drugs substantially reduces progression to acquired immunodeficiency syndrome (AIDS), hospitalization, opportunistic infections (OIs) and mortality. Recently released guidelines for HIV management have stressed on simplified regimens with fixed dose combinations to increase patient compliance.

BENEFITS OF EARLY START OF ART

Early initiation of anti-retro viral therapy (ART) may help in achieving the following goals:

It results in a significantly enhanced quality of life, reduces morbidity and mortality, reduces the viral load and has a sustained effect and restores immune function. Early initiation has been associated with an increase in the absolute CD4 cell count, improvement in the CD4/CD8 ratio, decrease in plasma viral load and improvement in immune status.

To achieve and sustain these benefits, ART should be able to suppress HIVRNA to the lowest levels possible (ideally < 50 copies/mL). As the level of plasma viral load is reduced, there is a 96% less risk of transmission to sexual partners.

ELIGIBILITY FOR ART

There have been various guidelines in the past about how to initiate ART. The eligibility criteria were based historically on CD4 cell counts (which were < 200, later pushed put up to 350 and then to 500 cells/mm^3). It is presently recommended to "treat-all" HIV-positive cases by the World Health Organization as well as the National AIDS Control Organisation of India.

Initiation of ART is to be done irrespective of the CD4 cell count, clinical stage of the disease and age of the patient. The need for ART by all HIV-positive patients means more medicines need to be manufactured and distributed to patients. It also means that AIDS-related death will sharply reduce. Thus, it is now a global policy that any HIV-positive individual should be placed on combination ART (cART).

When starting cART, the importance of adherence should be emphasized to the patient. Starting ART has been associated with a decreasedincidence of both AIDS-defining and non-AIDS-defining illnesses. It has also been associated with a higher life spend than in those in whom the initiating was done at a low CD4 cell count threshold.

HISTORY TAKING BEFORE INITIATION OF ART

Before starting ART, a good medical history regarding risk factors is important as it helps in counseling and providing support.

These risk factors are:

- Injectable drug abusers
- Commercial sex workers either male or female
- Men having sex with men
- History of unprotected sexual exposure especially with a commercial sex worker
- History of sexually transmitted diseases
- History of having received blood or blood products
- Injections, tattoos, ear piercing or body piercing using unsterile equipment.

BASELINE LABORATORY TESTS TO BE DONE BEFORE STARTING ART

Baseline laboratory tests include the following:

- CD4 cell count
- Complete blood count, alanine aminotransferase (ALT)/aspartate aminotransferase (AST), serum alkaline phosphatase, urine routine microscopy
- *For women*: Annual Pap smear screening
- Hepatitis B and hepatitis C screening for intravenous (IV) drug abusers
- Screening for tuberculosis (TB) at every visit
- Any other relevant investigations based on clinical signs and symptoms.

ART IN PREGNANT AND BREASTFEEDING WOMEN

Anti-retro viral therapy should be given to all pregnant and breastfeeding women diagnosed with HIV infection, irrespective of age, clinical stage, CD4 count. It should be continued lifelong.

TIMING OF ART INITIATION FOR ADULTS AND CHILDREN WITH TUBERCULOSIS

Anti-retro viral therapy should be started in all patients with TB and HIV regardless of their CD4 counts.

TB treatment should be started first, followed by ART as soon as possible within the first 8 weeks of treatment.

Among HIV-positive TB patients, those with CD4 counts less than 50 cells/ mm^3 should receive ART within the first 2 weeks of starting antituberculosis treatment (ATT).

ART IN PRESENCE OF OTHER OPPORTUNISTIC INFECTIONS

Anti-retro viral therapy should not be started in the presence of an active opportunistic infection. OIs should be treated first and the patient should be stabilized before initiating ART. Exceptions to these are *Mycobacterium avium* complex (MAC) and progressive multifocal leukoencephalopathy (PML), in which initiating ART is the mainstay of treatment (Table 6.1).

Table 6.1: Guidelines for initiation of anti-retro viral therapy.

	Old guidelines	*New guidelines*
If the CD 4 cellsare less than or equal to 500 cells/cmm^3	Yes	Not dependent of CD4 cell
WHO classical stage 3 or 4 or CD4 <350 cells/mm^3	Yes	All stages of illness
Malignancy	Yes	Yes
Elderly	Yes	Irrespective of age
Coinfection HBV/HCV	Yes	Yes
Coexisting tuberculosis	Yes	Within 8 weeks of ATT
Serodiscordant couples	No	Yes
Acute HIV	May be	Yes
All positive patients, irrespective of CD4 cell counts	No	Yes
Regardless of clinical stage of WHO	No	Yes
Pregnancy and breastfeeding women with HIV	Yes	Yes

WHEN TO START ART IN ADULTS AND ADOLESCENTS?

Table 6.2 gives details of opportunistic infection in HIV and when to start anti-retro viral therapy.

Table 6.2: When to start art in adults and adolescents.

Opportunistic infection	*Comment*	*ART therapy*
Cryptosporidium, Microsponidosis, Progressive multifocal leucoencephalopathy	These diseases do not have specific effective treatments. ART should be started as soon as possible to benefit the primary disease	As soon as possible
Pneumocystitis Jiovecui pneumonia	Immediate initiation of ART has been associated with increase survival	Immediate
Cryptococcal meningitis, tuberculosis		Short delay

CONCLUSION

- The goals of therapy are to improve the immune status of the patient, to reduce mortality or morbidity associated with HIV, to improve the quality of life of the person suffering from HIV/AIDS and to prevent further transmission of HIV.
- Early initiation of ART has been recommended in all guidelines.
- The START and TEMPRANO trials have provided recommendations about initiating ART in all positive patients irrespective of CD4 cell counts.
- Anti-retro viral therapy should be offered to all individuals who are at risk of transmitting HIV to their partners. However, it should be explained to the patient that ART is not a substitute for a condom as it does not protect against other venereal infections.
- During pregnancy, the goal should be plasma suppression of HIV. Perinatal transmission is markedly reduced by ART and should be offered to all pregnant women.
- Adherent to therapy should always be emphasized to the patient.

SUGGESTED READING

1. Abdool Karim SS, Naidoo K, Grobler A, et al. Timing of initiation of antiretroviral drugs during tuberculosis therapy. N Engl J Med. 2010;362(8):697-706.
2. Blanc FX, Sok T, Laureillard D, et al. Earlier versus later start of antiretroviral therapy in HIV-infected adul'ts with tuberculosis. N Engl J Med. 2011;365(16):1471-81.

3. Boulware DR, Meya DB, Muzoora C, et al. Timing of antiretroviral therapy after diagnosis of cryptococcal meningitis. N Engl J Med. 2014;370(26):2487-98.
4. Cain LE, Logan R, Robins JM, et al. When to initiate combined antiretroviral therapy to reduce mortality and AIDS-defining illness in HIV-infected persons in developed countries: an observational study. Ann Intern Med. 2011;154(8):509-15.
5. CASCADE Collaboration. Timing of HAART initiation and clinical outcomes in human immunodeficiency virus type 1 seroconverters. Arch Intern Med. 2011;171 (17):1560-69.
6. Cohen MS, Chen YQ, McCauley M, et al. Antiretroviral therapy for the prevention of HIV-1 transmission. N Engl J Med. 2016;375(9):830-9.
7. Havlir DV, Kendall MA, Ive P, et al. Timing of antiretroviral therapy for HIV-1 infection and tuberculosis. N Engl J Med. 2011;365(16):1482-91.
8. INSIGHT START Study Group, Lundgren JD, Babiker AG, et al. Initiation of antiretroviral therapy in early asymptomatic HIV infection. N Engl J Med. 2015;373 (9):795-807.
9. Kitahata MM, Gange SJ, Abraham AG, et al. Effect of early versus deferred antiretroviral therapy for HIV on survival. N Engl J Med. 2009;360(18):1815-26.
10. Palella FJJ, Armon C, Chmiel JS, et al. CD4 cell count at initiation of ART, long-term likelihood of achieving CD 4 >750 cells/mm3 and mortality risk. The Journal of antimicrobial chemotherapy. 2016;71(9):2654-62.
11. Severe P, Juste MA, Ambroise A, et al. Early versus standard antiretroviral therapy for HIV-infected adults in Haiti. N Engl J Med. 2010;363(3):257-65.
12. Sterne JA, May M, Costagliola D, et al. Timing of initiation of antiretroviral therapy in AIDS-free HIV-1-infected patients: a collaborative analysis of 18 HIV cohort studies. Lancet. 2009;373(9672):1352-63.
13. TEMPRANO ANRS Study Group, Danel C, Moh R, et al. A trial of early antiretrovirals and isoniazid preventive therapy in Africa. N Engl J Med. 2015;373(9):808-22.
14. Torok ME, Yen NT, Chau TT, et al. Timing of initiation of antiretroviral therapy in human immunodeficiency virus (HIV)—associated tuberculous meningitis. Clin Infect Dis. 2011;52(11):1374-83.

CHAPTER 7

What Anti-retro Viral Drugs to Start?

Atul Gogia, Parul Goel, Atul Kakar

INTRODUCTION

Once a patient is diagnosed as being HIV positive, the newer guidelines suggest starting anti-retro viral treatment (ART) as soon as possible. There are many groups of drugs presently available for the treatment of such patients and the selection depends upon the national guidelines, cost and their comorbid conditions (e.g. tuberculosis, anemia, hepatitis, etc.).

NATIONAL AIDS CONTROL ORGANIZATION (NACO) GUIDELINES

First-line Anti-retro Viral Treatment

According to the NACO guidelines, first-line ART should include two nucleoside reverse transcriptase inhibitors and one non-nucleoside reverse transcriptase inhibitor. These are to be started in ART naïve individuals after certain baseline clinical and laboratory tests.

These are:

1. CD4 cell count.
2. Complete blood count, aspartate transminase/alanine transminase (ALT/AST), serum alkaline phosphatase, serum creatinine, urine routine microscopy.
3. Annual PAP smear screening in women.
4. Hepatitis B and Hepatitis C screening for intravenous drug abusers.
5. Screening for tuberculosis at every visit.
6. Any other relevant investigations based on clinical signs and symptoms.

First-line Treatment Protocol (NACO Approved)

Clinical scenario I: Hemoglobin ≥ 9 g/dL and patient is not taking anti-tuberculosis treatment (ATT):

Zidovudine + Lamivudine + Nevirapine

Clinical scenario II: Hemoglobin < 9 g/dL and patient is not taking ATT:

Tenofovir + Lamivudine + Nevirapine

Clinical scenario III: Hemoglobin ≥ 9 g/dL and patient is on ATT:

Zidovudine + Lamivudine + Efavirenz

Clinical scenario IV: Hemoglobin < 9 gm/dL and patient is on ATT or/and Hepatitis B or Hepatitis C coinfection/pregnancy with no history of nevirapine intake:

Tenofovir + Lamivudine + Efavirenz

General Considerations

- Efavirenz should be replaced with Nevirapine in patients on ATT after 2 weeks of ATT completion.
- Nevirapine should be restarted after using a lead-in dose for 2 weeks, if it has been stopped for >2 weeks.
- If a patient presents with anemia after starting on Zidovudine-based therapy, then Zidovudine should be replaced with Tenofovir.
- In case of Tenofovir toxicity:
  - If the patient is not anemic, then Zidovudine is to be given
  - if the patient has anemia then Stavudine is to be used.
- Zidovudine should not be reintroduced in patients who have developed anemia due to the drug.
- Nevirapine should not be reintroduced in patients who have severe hypersensitivity (e.g. Stevens-Johnson syndrome and toxic epidermal necrolysis) to Nevirapine.

WHO RECOMMENDATIONS FOR ADULTS AND ADOLESCENTS

- According to the WHO also, first-line ART consists of two nucleoside reverse transcriptase inhibitors and one non-nucleoside reverse transcriptase inhibitor.
- A fixed dose combination is strongly recommended

  Lamivudine (or Emtricitabine) + Tenofovir + Efavirenz

- In case of non-availability of the above mentioned combination, or in the presence of any contraindication, suggested alternatives include the following:

  Zidovudine + Lamivudine + Efavirenz

  Zidovudine + Lamivudine + Nevirapine

  Tenofovir + Lamivudine (or Emtricitabine) + Nevirapine

WHO discourages the use of Stavudine in the first-line ART due to its metabolic toxicities.

ART IN PREGNANT AND BREASTFEEDING WOMEN

Anti-retro viral therapy should be given in all pregnant and breastfeeding women diagnosed with HIV infection, irrespective of age, clinical stage, CD4 count. It should also be continued lifelong. The details are given in another chapter.

ART IN THE PRESENCE OF OPPORTUNISTIC INFECTIONS

Anti-retro viral should not be started in the presence of an active opportunistic infections (OIs). OIs should be treated first and the patient stabilized before initiating ART. Exceptions to these are Mycobacterium Avium Complex (MAC) infection and progressive multifocal leukoencephalopathy (PML), in which initiating ART is the main stay of treatment.

FIRST-LINE ANTI-RETRO VIRAL TREATMENT FAILURE: FOLLOW-UP AND MONITORING

Patients on first-line ART should be monitored as per the following recommendations:

- At each visit, WHO staging for clinical events.
- Routine laboratory investigations, and CD4 cell count 6 monthly or earlier if needed.

High index of suspicion is required for identifying treatment failure.

After ensuring patient compliance for a minimum 6 months, failure of first line ART can be suspected in case of the following events:

- Slow or no improvement in the clinical condition of the patient.
- Appearance/recurrence of opportunistic infections or clinical events.
- Worsening of the patient clinically.
- Persistent decrease in the CD4 cell count.

OUTCOMES DURING THE FIRST SIX MONTHS OF THERAPY

The initial six months of ART are important. Although clinical and immunological improvement is expected complications are common in the first few weeks after the initiation in patients with severe immunodeficiency.

- *CD4 recovery*: The lower the baseline CD4 count at the start of ART, the longer will it take for the count to increase with time. In some patients although clinical improvement occurs, the count may never go beyond 200 cells/mm^3. In most patients however, the CD4 cell count rises with the initiation of ART.

- Early ART toxicity.
- *Mortality on ART*: While ART significantly decreases mortality; the risk of death is higher in the first six months than during the subsequent periods on therapy.
- *Immune reconstitution inflammatory syndrome (IRIS)*: This is a spectrum of clinical signs and symptoms resulting from the body's ability to mount an inflammatory response associated with immune recovery, occurrence or manifestations of new OIs or existing OIs within six weeks to six months after initiating ART; with an increase in CD4 count.

ART FAILURE DEFINITIONS

Clinical failure

WHO stage 4 developing or recurring even after 6 months of ART.

Immunological failure

- CD4 count declines to levels as before treatment
- CD4 count shows a decline of 50% from the peak value
- CD4 counts continue to be below 100 cells/uL.

Virological failure

Persistence of more than 5,000 copies/mL of virus in the plasma even after 6 months of anti-retro viral therapy.

Note:

- The above definitions are suggested by NACO.
- Possibility of IRIS should be excluded.
- Second line ART to be considered in case of some WHO stage 3 conditions which imply treatment failure (pulmonary Koch's, bacterial infections).
- Second line ART is not required in some WHO stage 4 conditions which do not imply treatment failure such as lymph node TB, pleural disease, esophageal candidiasis and recurrent bacterial pneumonia.
- Change of treatment should be considered only when the viral count is more than 5,000 cells/mm^3.

INTOLERANCE TO ZIDOVUDINE/TENOFOVIR AND NEVIRAPINE/EFAVIRENZ

Intolerance or toxicity or drug interactions require replacement of drugs in various groups.

- *Zidovudine and Tenofovir intolerance/toxicity*:

  Stavudine + Lamivudine + NNRTI (nevirapine or efavirenz)

- *Nevirapine and Efavirenz intolerance:* Atazanavir or low dose Ritonavir and continuing the previous NRTI (zidovudine/Tenofovir + Lamivudine).
- *Tenofovir, Zidovudine and Lamivudine intolerance*: Abacavir-based therapy.

SECOND-LINE ANTI-RETRO VIRAL TREATMENT

According to NACO guidelines, second-line ART is given after failure of first-line treatment.

Aim of second-line ART: Prolonged survival of People Living with HIV (PLHIV) by viral suppression for as long as possible.

NACO Second-line Regimen

Preferred Regimen

Tenofovir 300 mg + Lamivudine 300 mg + Atazanavir 300 mg/Ritonavir 100 mg

Clinical scenario I: Patients who showed toxicity to nevirapine and efavirenz/second-line therapy for patients who were on first-line ART having tenofovir with hemoglobin ≥ 9:

Zidovudine + Lamivudine + Atazanavir/Ritonavir

Clinical scenario II: Clinical scenario I patients who showed toxicity to Atazanavir/HIV-2 infection and Haemoglobin≥9 g/dl:

Zidovudine + Lamivudine + Lopinavir/Ritonavir

Clinical scenario III: Second-line treatment for patients with first-line ART having Zidovudine or Stavudine/patients with first-line ART having Tenofovir and who showed toxicity to Nevirapine and Efavirenz:

Tenofovir + Lamivudine + Atazanavir/Ritonavir

Clinical scenario IV: Clinical scenario III patients who showed toxicity to Atazanavir/HIV-2 infection and Hb < 9 g/dL/females with history of Nevirapine intake:

Tenofovir + Lamivudine + Lopinavir/Ritonavir

Clinical scenario V: Second-line therapy for patients with first-line ART having Tenofovir and hemoglobin < 9 g/dL:

Stavudine + Lamivudine + Atazanavir/Ritonavir

Clinical scenario VI: Clinical scenario V patients who showed toxicity to Atazanavir:

Stavudine + Lamivudine + Lopinavir/Ritonavir

To ensure patient compliance NACO advocates use of following tools:

- Patient counseling diary (individual)
- Use the Visual Analogue Scale (VAS) to help understand drug adherence
- Patient education information leaflets for their prescribed regimens
- Patient pill-taking monthly calendar.

COMMON NAMES OF SOME DRUG COMBINATIONS AVAILABLE IN MARKET

Drug combination	Brand name
Tenofovir + Emtricitabine + Efavirenz	Viraday (Cipla) Trustiva (Hetero) Teevir (Mylan)
Tenofovir + Lamivudine + Efavirenz	Trioday (Cipla) Tenolam E (Hetero) Tellura (Mylan)
Lamivudine + Nevirapine + Stavudine	Triomune (Cipla)
Tenofovir + Emtricitabine + Atazanavir/Ritonavir	Qvir kit (Cipla) Truvataz-R (Hetero)
Lamivudine + Zidovudine + Efavirenz	Duovir kit (Cipla)
Lamivudine + Zidovudine + Nevirapine	Duovir N kit (Cipla) Zidolam-N (Hetero)

CONCLUSION

- There are many regimes for treatment of HIV/AIDS. After discussion with the patient about cost, compliance issues should also be discussed before starting ART.
- The adverse effects of ART could be mild, moderate to severe or life-threatening. Whereas mild side-effects do not require discontinuation of medicines, a change in ART is required in moderate to severe side-effects. In case of life-threatening toxicity (like Stevens-Johnson syndrome), discontinuation of ART is required till the patient is stabilized.
- Regular monitoring of the patient is required for early pick up of first line ART failure.

  A rational based regime should be initiated in all patients to achieve maximum viral suppression so that prolonged survival can be achieved.

SUGGESTED READING

1. Cohen MS, Chen YQ, Gamble T, et al. Prevention of HIV-1 infection with early antiretroviral therapy. N Engl J Med. 2011;365:493-505.
2. Kanters S, Socias ME, Paton NI, et al. Comparative efficacy and safety of second-line antiretroviral therapy for treatment of HIV/AIDS: a systematic review and network meta-analysis. The Lancet HIV. 2017;4(10):e433-41.
3. Kitahata MM, Gange SJ, Abraham AG, et al. Effect of early versus deffered antiretroviral therapy for HIV on survival. N Engl J Med. 2009;360:1815-26.
4. Lundgren JD, Babiker AG, Gordin F, et al. Initiation of antiretroviral therapy in early asymptomatic HIV infection. N Engl J Med. 2015; 373:795-807.

5. Mallolas J. Darunavir stands up as preferred HIV protease inhibitor. AIDS Reviews. 2017;19(2):105-12.
6. Olding M, Enns B, Panagiotoglou D, et al. A historical review of HIV prevention and care initiatives in British Columbia, Canada: 1996-2015. J Int AIDS Soc. 2017;20(1):21941.
7. Severe P, Amroise A, Eliasin L, et al. Early versus standard antiretroviral therapy for HIV-infected adults in Haiti. N Engl J Med. 2010;363:257-65.
8. WHO. Guideline on when to start antiretroviral therapy and on pre-exposure prophylaxis for HIV. September, 2015. Available from www.who.int/hiv/pub/guidelines/earlyrelease-arv/en.

CHAPTER 8

How to Monitor Anti-retro Viral Therapy?

Jyoti Kotwal

Patients living with human immunodeficiency virus (HIV)/acquired immunodeficiency syndrome (AIDS) [PLHA] have to be monitored as part of their chronic care while on treatment with anti-retro viral therapy (ART). The monitoring involves both clinical and laboratory methods. The CD4 cells are asubset of T lymphocytes and are destroyed by the HIV as they are its primary target. The decrease in CD4 cells causes the immune response to weaken thus rendering the patient susceptible to infections which leads to the development of AIDS. Patients can also have coinfections with the hepatitis B and hepatitis C viruses. Screening for these infections has to be done as the choice of ART is changed and also monitoring for these coinfections is mandatory while on therapy.

As the disease is a viral disease and affects the immune system monitoring of patients for response to therapy is basically observing the immunological and virological response in the patient. However, monitoring of the side effects of therapy, ART-associated allergic reactions and HIV resistance assays are equally important.

Many laboratory tests are done for the initial evaluation and follow-up of HIV-infected patients on ART to assess the immunological and efficacy of the ART as well as to monitor anti-retro viral (ARV) drugs.

Two markers that are routinely used to monitor them are:

1. CD4 T-lymphocyte cell count to assess immune function.
2. Plasma HIV RNA to assess the level of HIV virus load in the patient. HIV-related illness progression and mortality is closely linked with the CD4 cell count and HIV viral load (RNA level). Progressive depletion of CD4+ T cells is associated with an increased chance of severe HIV disease and a poorer prognosis. This also provides information on the response to therapy and progression of the disease. Thus, both these tests are important in monitoring an HIV-positive individual on therapy.

Till recently, an absolute CD4 count of less than 350 cells/μL was used as a cutoff for initiation of ART in India and other resource-restricted countries in patients classified as the World Health Organization (WHO) clinical stage I and II while all patients with clinical stage III and IV had to be given on ART. Recently the WHO revised its recommendation and stated that irrespective of their CD4 cell counts all positive patients should receive treatment. This recommendation has also been accepted by the National AIDS Control Organization (NACO) of India.

LATEST RECOMMENDATIONS FOR CD4 MONITORING WHEN ON TREATMENT

The absolute CD4 count has to be used for monitoring disease activity at 3- to 6-month intervals. It should be repeated 3 months after the start of therapy and then every 4 months until the CD4 is greater than 200 cells/μL on two occasions at least 4 months apart and then monitored according to the specific situation. If the CD4 count increases to less than or equal to 300 cells/μL (between 200 and 300), then at least every 6 monthly testing is required. If the CD4 is between greater than 300 cells/μL and less than or equal to 500 cells/μL, 12 monthly monitoring is recommended. If CD4 greater than 500 cells/μL, then further monitoring becomes optional, if the individual is asymptomatic. If, while on therapy there is a fall in CD4 count then it implies that either there is improper adherence or the development of resistance to therapy. According to the literature, an increase in CD4 cell counts greater than 200/μL is an indicator of success of therapy. Also, severe opportunistic infections (OIs) can a cause fall in the CD4 countless than 200/μL. Thus, a cutoff of CD4 count of less than 200 cells/μL is very important in follow-up. A CD4 countless than 200/μL is an indicator to start prophylaxis against *Pneumocystis jirovecii* pneumonia. A CD4 count of less than 50 cells/μL means that there is a likelihood to get *Mycobacterium avium* complex infection and prophylaxis against it is required. If the CD4 count greater than 200 cells/μL prophylaxis against OIs can be stopped as it implies a good response to the ART.

Good response criteria are—a CD4 count increase of greater than 50 cells/μL within 4–8 weeks after the viral suppression has occurred. It should then increase by 50–100 cells/μL/year. In some cases, CD4 counts may not increase quickly or steadily, even after good viral load suppression. This is typically seen in older patients (age >50 years) or in those who had lower baseline CD4 cell counts at the start of therapy.

Practically, both in stable untreated patients and in patients on ART, the CD4 count should be repeated approximately every 3–6 months. For patients on ART who have persistently suppressed HIV RNA and have CD4 counts continuously above thresholds for OI risk (>200 cells/μL); the current guidelines suggest monitoring every 6–12 months. The CD4 count should be checked more often if indicated (e.g. in patients after change of ART, those with ART failure and those with rapidly declining CD4 counts).

Measuring the CD4 count and CD4 percentage: The measurement is done in flow cytometer and the test should be done ideally within 24 hours of collecting the blood sample in an ethylenediaminetetraacetic acid (EDTA) tube. The test can be done on a double platform where the percentage of CD4 cells of all lymphocytes is assessed on a flow cytometer and the absolute lymphocyte count (ALC) from the cell counter. The CD4 count is then calculated from the CD4 percentage and ALC. The more accurate method is the single platform technique, where the absolute CD4 count, CD8 count and the ratio are calculated on the flow cytometer. Here calibrating beads and/or Trucount tubes are used. This is the recommended method by the WHO and a sample report by this method, as done in our laboratory, is given later in the text. The CD4 count should ideally be done only in a NACO or National Accreditation Board for Testing and Calibration Laboratories (NABL)—approved laboratory to get accurate and reliable results.

The normal values for CD4 count vary considerably among different laboratories. The mean normal value for most laboratories is approximately 300–1,400 CD4 cells/μL. This is subject to slight fluctuations. Diurnal, illness, vaccination variation and laboratory error can result in transient CD4 cell count changes. A CD4 percentage of less than 14% is considered to correspond to the same degree of immunosuppression as an absolute CD4 count of less than 200 cells/μL. As CD4 counts can vary, clinical decisions generally should not be made on the basis of a single value. If the results are inconsistent, the test should be repeated, and treatment decisions usually should be based on two or more similar values. A change is significant if there is a 30% change in absolute CD4 count or CD4 percentage changes by 3%. Additionally, the CD4:CD8 ratio can also be assessed.

Immunological failure is defined as a 50% fall from on treatment peak value of the CD4 value or persistent CD4 values less than 100/μL while on therapy.

RECOMMENDATIONS FOR HIV VIRAL LOAD MONITORING

- For patients starting on ART.
- Those changing therapy as a result of virological failure.

The HIV RNA should be measured 4 weeks after the initiation of therapy and is reported as copies of the virus/mL of blood sample. If the therapy is effective, there should be a dip by at least 1 log (10-fold) in the viral load. For patients who do not have pre-existent ARV resistance, an undetectable viral load (<50 copies/mL) is usually achieved within 3 months. Patients with an

HIV viral load greater than 100,000 copies/mL at baseline should achieve an undetectable viral load within 6 months of effective treatment. If this does not happen, it suggests resistance to the ARV drugs being administered.

If the viral load response to ART is absent or incomplete, it should alert physician about poor adherence to therapy and/or viral resistance.

If a patient who has had suppression of viral load while on ART gets detectable viral values between 40 copies/mL and 500 copies/mL, it is not virological failure but most probably a low-level transient presence of the virus in the blood (transient viremia). This is also called a blip. A blip means that there is a transient increase in the viral copy numbers/mL in a suppressed patient and when a repeat test is done the viral copy numbers (viral load) are again below the level of detectable by quantitative polymerase chain reaction (PCR) on repeat testing performed promptly after a positive result. However, a persistent elevation, even at low levels, is not a blip and needs further investigation. Recent vaccination and/or an acute concurrent illness may cause this transient rise. Blips do not require a change in ART as they are not known to be associated with the development of resistance mutations or virological failure. Retesting should be ordered after 4 weeks to differentiate a blip from virological failure. Thus, ART should not be changed based on a single viral load elevation.

Viral treatment failure: A persistent rise in the viral load indicates viral failure. The optimal viral load threshold for determining virological failure has not been validated. Persistent viral copies greater than 5,000 copies/mL are associated with clinical progression with decline in the CD4 cell count. This can be thus taken as an indicator of treatment failure.

Real-time PCR technology is widely used for HIV-1 RNA quantification. This is also called Quantitative- or Rq-PCR. The currently available HIV-1 viral load tests use real-time PCR technology which offersa larger dynamic range of quantification than earlier viral load tests. The lower and upper limits of quantification of the currently available the US Food and Drug Administration (FDA)-approved HIV-1 viral load tests are 25–50 copies/mL and 10,000,000 copies/mL, respectively. Several different HIV viral load tests have been developed, and four are currently approved are:

1. Abbott RealTime HIV-1 (Abbott Laboratories)
2. Cobas AmpliPrep/Cobas TaqMan HIV-1 Test, version 2.0 (Roche Diagnostics)
3. Cobas HIV-1 quantitative NAT for use on Cobas 6800/8800 systems (Roche Diagnostics)
4. Cobas TaqMan HIV-1 Test, v2.0 for use with the high pure system (Roche Diagnostics)

As this test is not available with most hospital laboratories in India due to the cost benefits of doing only a few samples, it is usually outsourced. It is important to understand which are the approved tests, soonly proper testing in proper laboratories is done for monitoring the patients.

Immunological or viral failure: This is an indication to change the ART therapy and is an ART switching criteria. It is at this time that resistance studies of the virus to drugs need to be done in a research laboratory to decide on the alternative second-line ART to be given. Failure to respond to a recommended ART regimen is almost always a result of suboptimal adherence or viral resistance.

Adherence monitoring: It is a very important part of monitoring a patient on therapy. At each visit, patients should be interviewed regarding medication adherence in a nonjudgmental manner by the doctor. The patient's relatives should also monitor adherence in a subtle way. Education of the patient and his or her family on the importance of adherence is very important. Nonadherence can cause progression of disease as well as development of resistance of the virus to the first-line drugs which the patient is on. Understanding that nonadherence will lead to drug resistance and thus disease progression is very important for all patients on treatment.

LABORATORY MONITORING OF ART SIDE EFFECTS

Anti-retro viral therapy can lead to some side effects in some patients like bone marrow suppression, pancreatitis, hepatotoxicity, an abnormal lipid profile and renal toxicity.

Complete blood counts [consisting of hemoglobin (Hb), total white blood cell (WBC) count, differential leukocyte count (DLC) and platelet count] should be measured before initiation of therapy and every 4 months thereafter for *bone marrow suppression* monitoring. However, in patients with a high risk of bone marrow toxicity (e.g. those with advanced HIV infection, those with pre therapy low counts or those receiving zidovudine), blood counts need to be monitored more frequently (every month), as the counts may fall drastically in them.

Pancreatitis should be considered in any patient receiving ART who presents with signs or symptoms like abdominal pain, persistent nausea, and vomiting. Serum amylase and lipase should be obtained when this occurs.

Hypertriglyceridemia (triglycerides >500 mg/dL) is associated with an increased risk of pancreatitis, particularly in patients with other risk factors (e.g. alcohol or obesity/gallstones).

Thus, a 6 monthly monitoring of the lipid profile is recommended.

All ARV agents have the potential to cause abnormalities in liver function, especially in patients with pre-existing liver disease. Serum liver enzyme levels should be obtained at baseline and every 3–4 months in patients receiving ART. If a patient had a pre-existing liver disease or serum liver enzyme abnormalities, then 2 monthly liver function test (LFT) should be done. A higher incidence of significant hepatotoxicity has recently been reported with nevirapine therapy, especially in women and in the setting of hepatitis C virus coinfection. Such patients need to be monitored monthly for liver function while on therapy.

The HIV infection itself can cause renal complications that may lead to renal insufficiency or failure. Renal impairment may necessitate dose adjustment or discontinuation of many ARV agents. Thus, renal function (serum creatinine and blood urea) needs to be monitored 6 monthly and urine analysis should be done annually in a HIV patient on ART.

Renal impairment has been reported in patients receiving tenofovir and they also need to get regular renal function tests done 3 monthly.

MONITORING FOR ART-ASSOCIATED ALLERGIC REACTIONS

Many medications can cause a maculopapular rash, with or without feveras allergic reactions. Occasionally, a more severe hypersensitivity reaction occurs, and usually occurs within 2–6 weeks after the drug is started. Allergic reaction consist of fever, rash and other symptoms, such as headache, joint pains, jaundice, increased eosinophil count, wheezing and nausea and vomiting.

Trimethoprim/sulfamethoxazole given to prevent OIs is the most common cause of drug-induced allergic reactions in HIV/AIDS cases. Drugs like abacavir, darunavir, tipranavir, fosamprenavir, and all of the non-nucleoside reverse transcriptase inhibitors (NNRTIs) (nevirapine, delavirdine, efavirenz, etravirine), can cause a hypersensitivity reaction or hypersensitivity syndrome. These reactions are idiosyncratic and thus unanticipated. Sulfa-containing ART (darunavir, fosamprenavir, tipranavir) can cause mild to moderate skin allergy also called a drug rash. Patients may rarely develop severe mucous membrane involvement with systemic toxicity. Occasionally, patients can have only fever (drug fever). The treating physicians should consider the possibility of these reactions when the patients are put on ART because they are most commonly seen in the first 4 weeks of treatment. Education of patients about the symptoms of hypersensitivity helps in early detection of these reactions which can be treated by antiallergic drugs like Avil.

Discontinuation of abacavir is recommended when a hypersensitivity reaction is suspected. Once abacavir has been discontinued because of a possible or definite hypersensitivity reaction, it should never be administered again. Rechallenge may result in an anaphylactic reaction with associated hypotension or death. When a patient has to be put on abacavir-based therapy, HLA-B*5701 should be tested, and the drug should not be given if it is positive.

Nevirapine, an NNRTI, can cause severe hypersensitivity reactions in the first 2–12 weeks of use. Graduated dosing of nevirapine has reduced the incidence of hypersensitivity reactions. Some patients can develop a severe cutaneous reaction involving the mucocutaneous surfaces (Stevens-Johnson syndrome), which is accompanied with fever and severe hepatitis. This can be fatal if not detected in time. Mild rashes without systemic toxicity should be managed with antihistamines and close monitoring. The nevirapine dose should not be escalated to twice daily until the rash has resolved. Those patients with moderate to severe cutaneous toxicity should discontinue nevirapine promptly and should never be rechallenged with this drug. Because of likely cross-reactivity, use of an alternate NNRTI should be avoided in patients who have a severe reaction to nevirapine.

SURROGATE MARKERS FOR CD4 COUNT

In many resource-constrained countries, CD4 count is not readily available. In India, with the introduction of cheap generic drugs for ART, the therapy is available to all patients but they cannot afford the recommended 3–6 monthly CD4 counts. From our center, data of 2004–2005 was published addressing the issue of surrogate markers to predict CD4 count less than 200/μL and it was found that an ALC of less than or equal to 1,520/μL was a good indicator of CD4 cell count of less than or equal to 200/μL. However, this data is not applicable in the present scenario, as it was done by the less accurate double platform for CD4 estimation and was on ART-naïve patients and ART is now recommended for all cases. Thus, last year we published our data on surrogate markers on cell counters which may predict a critically low CD4 count at diagnosis or a fall in CD4 count less than 200/μL while on ART therapy. We found that an ALC obtained by a 5-part cell counter less than 1,250/μL is predictive of a CD4 count less than 200/μL with a sensitivity and specificity of 87.3% and 70.0%, respectively. Along with this, an Hb value less than 11.15g/dL is also a good predictor of the CD4 count less than 200/μL. The combination of both Hb less than 11.15 g/dL and ALC counter less than 1,250/μL was like a confirmatory test with a high specificity. We thus found a combination of Hb and ALCs obtained on automated cell counter to be accurate, cost-effective and easily available methods to follow-up PLHA patients on therapy. These can effectively predict the CD4 count less than 200/μL and are especially useful in a developing country where the cost of these tests is one-fifth of that of flow cytometry.

Table 8.1: Format of report of CD4 counts.

	Gating done on CD45+ cells			
			*Reference ranges**	
	Percentage	*Cells/µL*	*%*	*Cells/µL*
CD3-positive cells	74.24	456	60–90%	619–2,525
CD4-positive cells	12.80	79	32–68%	286–1,316
CD8-positive cells	60.55	372	10–36%	130–1,118
CD4/CD8 ratio	0.21		0.33–2.47	

Thus, we recommend that in PLHAs, routine monitoring may be done only by ALC and Hb determined on automated cell counters and values less than 1,250/µL and less than 11.15 g/dL, respectively be taken as warning signs of progression of disease/failure of therapy. Then the expensive CD4 estimation and viral load studies should be done. We recommend that CD4 counting may be restricted to patients fulfilling the above criteria. This may further mandate a workup for OIs and alternative ART.

Format of Report of CD4 Counts

- *Total leukocyte count*: 8.400/µL.
- *Absolute lymphocyte count*: 614/µL.

The format of report of CD4 counts has been shown in Table 8.1.

Comments

This is a single platform approach using CYTO-STAT tetra CHROME™ CD45-FITC/CD56-RD1/CD19-ECD/CD3-PC5 monoclonal antibody reagent and the Flow-Count Fluorosphere™ beads in 1:1 ratio with whole blood specimen. Immunoprep™ (Beckman Coulter, Fullerton, California, USA) reagent is used for red cell lysis and no washing is performed. By this procedure, values of ALC (ALC FCM), CD3%, absolute CD3 count, CD4%, absolute CD4 count, CD8%, absolute CD8 count and CD4:CD8 ratio is determined for all samples. The absolute counts were determined using the following formula:

$$\frac{\left(\begin{array}{c}\text{Total no. of cells of}\\ \text{interest counted}\end{array} \times \begin{array}{c}\text{Flowcount fluorospheres}\\ \text{assayed concentration}\end{array}\right)}{\left(\begin{array}{c}\text{Total no. of Flowcount}\\ \text{fluorospheres counted}\end{array}\right)}$$

The data from the flow cytometer for CD4 estimation in our lab with normal values has been shown in Figure 8.1.

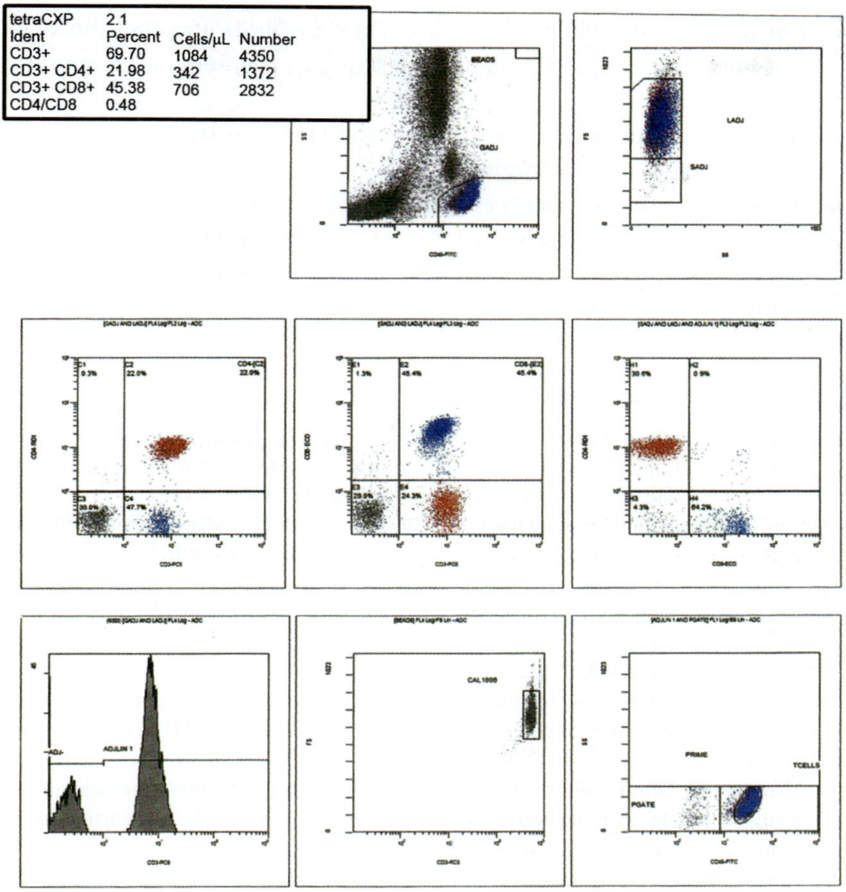

Fig. 8.1: Flow cytometry-based CD4 estimation.

CONCLUSION

- The CD4 cell count is the best indicator of the immune status and for determining whether a person is at risk of infection with certain OIs. The higher the CD4 count, the stronger the immune system.
- CD4 counts are variable. A physician should not change therapy based on a single laboratory result. A change of less than 30% in the CD4 count may not be clinically significant.
- The HIV viral load is the best indicator of the level of HIV activity in the patient's body.
- The goal of therapy is to suppress the viral load to below the detectable level by laboratory tests. However, an undetectable viral load does not mean HIV has been completely eradicated or that the patient is not infectious to others.

- For patients on ART, a rise in the CD4 count indicates that the virus has been suppressed. It also indicates an improvement in the immune system.
- In stable patients on ART, the CD4 count and HIV viral load usually should be monitored every 3–6 months.
- The ALC on the five-part cell counter is a surrogate indicator of CD4 counts and a value less than 1,250/μL is a danger sign and calls for a CD4 count in those with limited resources, not doing regular CD4 estimation.

SUGGESTED READING

1. AIDS Research Advisory Council (OARAC). (2017). Guidelines for the use of antiretroviral agents in HIV-1-infected adults and adolescents. [online] Available from https://aidsinfo.nih.gov/guidelines. [Accessed October 2017].
2. Anti-retroviral therapy guidelines for HIV-infected adults and adolescents. National AIDS Control Organization, Ministry of Family Welfare, Government of India, May 2013.
3. Buscher A, Mugavero M, Westfall AO, et al. The association of clinical follow-up intervals in HIV-infected persons with viral suppression on subsequent viral suppression. AIDS Patient Care STDs. 2013;27:459-66.
4. Gale HB, Gitterman SR, Hoffman HJ, et al. Is frequent CD4+ T-lymphocyte count monitoring necessary for persons with counts ≥300 cells/μL and HIV-1 suppression? Clin Infect Dis. 2013;56:1340-3.
5. Grennan JT, Loutfy MR, Su D, et al. Magnitude of virologic blips is associated with a higher risk for virologic rebound in HIV-infected individuals: a recurrent events analysis. J Infect Dis. 2012;205:1230-8.
6. Kotwal J, Dass J, Kotwal A, et al. Evaluation of surrogate markers for prediction of CD4 counts in people living with human immunodeficiency virus/acquired immunodeficiency syndrome. J AIDS Clin Res. 2016;7:573.
7. Romih V, ZidovecLepej S, Gedike K, et al. Frequency of HIV-1 viral load monitoring of patients initially successfully treated with combination antiretroviral therapy. PLoS One. 2010;5:e15051.

SECTION 4

Women and HIV

CHAPTER
9

Management of Mother-to-Child Transmission of HIV

Chandra Mansukhani, Rashmi Nigam

INTRODUCTION

Pregnancy accompanied by a human immunodeficiency virus (HIV) infection requires multidisciplinary care. Prevention of this HIV infection is an important concern, and to prevent vertical transmission, all testing for HIV infection in pregnant women is an ideal practice. In most of the developed countries, the rate of HIV infection transmission from mother to child has declined to very low levels (<2%) with the use of multidrug anti-retro viral therapy (ART), scheduled Cesarean section, avoidance of breastfeeding and 6 weeks of zidovudine prophylaxis for infants. In some developing countries, a significant reduction in HIV transmission to the child has also been reported with simple and short courses of anti-retro viral regimen and exclusive breastfeeding for 6 months.

In developing countries, women in the reproductive age group are at risk of seroconversion. In 2015, worldwide there were an estimated 17.8 million women living with HIV, which constitute 51% of all adults with HIV. Many women are diagnosed for the first time during pregnancy. Mother-to-child transmission in non-breastfeeding European women is 15–20% and 25–40% in breastfeeding Africans. Transmission during pregnancy, during labor and in the postpartum period can be reduced significantly by multidrug ART and avoiding breastfeeding. Available therapies, monotherapy as well as combined ART (three or more drugs) has dramatically reduced the morbidity and mortality, increased the lifespan and prevented vertical as well as horizontal transmission.

PRENATAL COUNSELING

- All newly diagnosed HIV-positive women should have an early initial evaluation of their social condition and they should be assured about its confidentiality.

- All pregnant females visiting antenatal clinics should be tested for HIV after obtaining informed written consent and being allowed to opt out from testing.
- The main aim of the prenatal or preconceptional counseling is to identify and reduce the high risk of adverse factors for maternal, fetal and couple health.
- The patient and her partner should be counseled regarding the worsening of any existing disease and the condition of the mother, the need of ART for improving their health and how to prevent vertical transmission of infection to the baby.
- A couple desiring a child should be counseled about the present status of the infection, the ideal timing of conception and the management of the pregnancy.

Couples should be offered the option of medical termination of pregnancy (MTP), if they are not ready to take or are unable to afford ART. The couple should be explained about the disadvantages of high-risk behavior, which would further increase the risk of perinatal transmission. Counseling should also include abstaining from cigarette smoking, drug use (e.g. cocaine, heroin) and unprotected sexually intercourse with multiple partners. If both partners are HIV-positive, counseling should be done regarding the risk of super added sexually transmitted infections associated with unprotected sex. Among HIV serodiscordant couples, the consistent use of condoms reduces the risk of HIV transmission by 80%.

DIAGNOSIS

Testing Guidelines

- Routine antenatal HIV testing in the first trimester is strongly recommended for every pregnant woman. If the test is negative, repeat HIV testing should be considered in the third trimester in high prevalence areas, especially for women with high-risk behavior. Women presenting in labor for the first time should undergo rapid HIV testing. Those with a positive rapid test should be started on prophylaxis till confirmatory tests are available.

Tests

- The recommended first-line antenatal HIV tests are presently the fourth-generation ones. They use enzyme immunoassays for antibodies against HIV-1 (M and O), HIV-2 as well as the p24 antigen test which remains the only marker during the window period of the infection. This period typically may range from 3 weeks to 6 months from infection to seroconversion (production of measurable antibodies to the HIV). Reaction assays are retested twice independently to increase their specificity.

- Positive tests are then forwarded for confirmation, i.e. a Western blot or immunofluorescent assays. If the Western blot returns on e-band of each GAG, POL and ENV gene product groups, the test is considered positive. Western blot is a test of HIV proteins that are produced by recombinant DNA to RNA of the virus by recombinant immunoblot assay (RIBA).
- Some centers offer a third-generation assay that tests for HIV-1/2 but not for the p24 antigen, therefore missing the initial infection that may have happened during the window period.

Rapid or Point-of-Care Tests

- Rapid tests give the results within 20 minutes. A sample can be taken by a finger prick or an oral swab. These tests do not test for the p24 antigen but only for antibodies to HIV-1 and 2 and are primarily used for unbooked patients presenting in late antenatal period or in active labor. There is a high false-positive rate with oral swabs and finger-pricks; therefore, whole blood is a better sample.

EFFECT OF HIV ON THE COURSE AND OUTCOME OF PREGNANCY

- *Poor pregnancy outcome*: There are increased chances of first trimester pregnancy loss and the chances of ectopic pregnancy are higher with HIV infection.
- *Small for gestational age*: There are greater chances of small for gestational age in pregnancy in mothers infected with HIV, hence serial growth scans should be done especially in the third trimester to assess the development of the intrauterine growth rate (IUGR) and decide the management accordingly.
- *Preterm birth*: There is an increased risk of preterm delivery prior to 37 weeks of gestation in HIV-positive pregnant women on combination therapy containing protease inhibitors but, given the clear benefits to maternal health and reduction in perinatal transmission of HIV, a protease inhibitor-based combination anti-retro viral regimen remains the recommendation for HIV-infected pregnant women.

FACTORS WHICH INCREASE THE RISK OF VERTICAL TRANSMISSION OF HIV

- In developing countries, it is estimated that every minute a child is infected with HIV as a result of transmission during the antenatal, intranatal and postnatal periods, which is potentially preventable. In India, approximate 1.8–2.9 million people are living with HIV, and of these 39% are women of reproductive age with a national average antenatal prevalence of 0.48%.

- Factors affecting transmission include maternal, viral, obstetric and fetal factors.
- The risk of vertical transmission increases with factors such as seroconversion during pregnancy, advanced stage of disease, maternal malnutrition and high maternal viral load.
- The concomitant presence of sexually transmitted disease (STD) and/or suboptimal ART increases the risk of mother-to-child transmission.
- The risk factors which would increase the transmission during the intrapartum period are mode of delivery, prolonged rupture of membranes and prolonged contact of the fetus with maternal blood/cervicovaginal secretions. Maternal chorioamnionitis and invasive procedures like fetal scalp electrode insertion or instrumental delivery also increase the transmission of HIV to the fetus.
- Premature fetuses are at an increased risk of vertical transmission because of susceptible mucous membranes, an immature fetal immune system and the presence of low levels of maternal antibodies.
- In the postnatal period, risk factors include breastfeeding, mixed feeding, feeding with cracked nipples/mastitis, a high viral load in the mother and a low CD4 count.
- In the absence of any ART intervention, the rate of mother-to-child transmission is very high, i.e. 15–30% in the developed countries and 30–45% in developing countries. This difference is mainly because of breastfeeding for a prolonged duration and mixed feeding.

ANTENATAL EVALUATION

Pregnant women with HIV infection should be managed by a multidisciplinary approach which includes an HIV physician, obstetrician, specialist midwife, health adviser and pediatrician. Comprehensive medical care of HIV-infected pregnant women is usually associated with favorable maternal health outcomes and low rates of perinatal HIV transmission.

HISTORY AND PHYSICAL EXAMINATION

- A detailed history and physical examination should be performed for every HIV-positive pregnant woman to assess the stage of the disease and rule out any pre-existing medical disorder which may affect the well-being of the fetus and increase the risk of perinatal transmission.
- A detailed history should be taken regarding the presence of opportunistic infection, tuberculosis, STDs, any specific medication use, immunization status and substance abuse.
- The nutritional status of every pregnant woman should be evaluated to rule out anemia and vitamin deficiencies as the poor nutritional status of the mother increases the risk of vertical transmission.

- A detailed physical examination should be done for every patient to look for the presence of any signs of advanced HIV infection (e.g. oral thrush or evidence of wasting) or signs of concomitant STDs (e.g. genital ulcers or vaginal discharge). Annual cervical cytology is recommended for all HIV-infected pregnant or nonpregnant women for diagnosis of cervical neoplasia as there is a strong correlation between HIV, human papillomavirus (HPV) infections and cervical neoplasia.
- A careful examination should be carried out for stigmata of advanced liver disease, e.g. hepatomegaly, splenomegaly and spider angiomata as HIV-infected patients are at a higher risk for viral hepatitis.

MANAGEMENT OF PREGNANCY WITH HIV INFECTION

This can be divided broadly in three parts, i.e. (1) antenatal, (2) intranatal and (3) postnatal management.

Antenatal Management

The main goal of antenatal management is to improve maternal health, give appropriate immunization, treat opportunistic infections or STDs, and prevent antepartum vertical transmission.

All HIV-infected pregnant women should have routine antenatal care (ANC) according to the National AIDS Control Organization (NACO) protocol, as described here.

- Every patient should have these minimum ANC checkups during pregnancy—the 1st visit should be within the first 12 weeks, the 2nd between 14 weeks and 26 weeks, the 3rd between 28 weeks and 32 weeks and the 4th between 36 weeks and 40 weeks as per the Reproductive and Child Health Programme (RCH)/National AIDS Control Programme (NACP) guidelines.
- A detailed history should be taken and a physical and abdominal examination should be done.
- Antenatal blood testing includes the following:
    - A complete blood count, blood group and Rh typing, routine urine examination at the 1st visit and tests for syphilis, hepatitis B, hepatitis C and HIV
    - A hemoglobin and urine examination should be done at all visits.
- Maternal immunization:
    - Two doses of tetanus toxoid (TT)
        - *First dose*: At the time of registration
        - *Second dose*: 4–6 weeks after the first dose

- Hepatitis B, pneumococcal, influenza vaccines—safely considered in unvaccinated pregnant women
- Rubella, measles, mumps (live vaccines)—to be deferred till delivery in immunoglobulin G (IgG)-negative patients.

- Antenatal drug supplementation:
  - Iron folic acid tablet (100 mg iron + 0.5 mg folic acid) everyday for 100 days, after the first trimester to prevent anemia
  - Double the dose if there is no rise in hemoglobin level.
- Treatment of opportunistic infections:
  - Appropriate treatment of STDs
  - Discordant and concordant couples—encouraged to use condoms consistently with sexual activity—as STDs can lead to preterm delivery and teratogenicity (e.g. congenital syphilis)
  - Routine testing for tuberculosis and if required ATT can be started
  - *Pneumocystis carinii* pneumonia (PCP) prophylaxis
    - *Prenatal period*: Cotrimoxazole
    - *First trimester*: Aerosolized pentamidine preferred
    - *Second and third trimester*: Cotrimoxazole (trimethoprim and sulfamethoxazole) and double strength daily/one single strength daily (better tolerated)/one double strength thrice weekly. Or alternatively Dapsone can be given.

Monitoring during Pregnancy

- First trimester dating scan to confirm gestational age.
- Second trimester anomaly scan to rule out teratogenic effects of ART.
- Plasma HIV viral load at 1st visit, 2–4 weeks after initiating or changing ART and then monthly till RNA levels are undetectable. RNA levels are then repeated every 3 months during pregnancy and at 36–37 weeks of gestation to plan for mode of delivery.
- CD4 T-lymphocyte counts are monitored at the 1st visit and then once in every trimester or after 3 months during pregnancy. Six-monthly monitoring can be done in patients who have been on ART for more than 2–3 years with good compliance and have sustained viral suppression.
- Rest of the monitoring of pregnancy for mother and fetus remains the same as that of a non-HIV-infected pregnant woman.

Prevention of Mother-to-Child Transmission of HIV

- Perinatal HIV infection transmission can occur during the antepartum, intrapartum or postpartum periods.
- However, with appropriate ART prophylaxis and effective viral suppression, the risk of perinatal transmission has become even less than 2% in the United States and Europe.

Thus combination ART is recommended for all pregnant HIV-infected women, regardless of CD4 T-lymphocyte count or plasma HIV RNA copy number, to prevent perinatal HIV transmission.

Clinical trials on prevention of HIV vertical transmission: In the year 1994, an AIDS clinical trial (Protocol 076) was conducted in the United States and France. This trial showed a significantly lower rate of perinatal transmission in patients who were on zidovudine (25% vs 8%) therapy.

Criteria for ART Initiation

Anti-retro viral therapy should be initiated early in pregnant women for her own health and to prevent transmission of HIV infection to her fetus.

The NACO recommendations for initiating ART in HIV-positive pregnant women are:

- Initiate lifelong ART in all pregnant women with confirmed HIV infection regardless of the World Health Organization (WHO) clinical stage or CD4 cell count.
- TDF+3TC+EFV is recommended as first-line ART in pregnant and breastfeeding women (even in the first trimester of pregnancy and women of childbearing age).

The alternate regimen if the pregnant women are unable to tolerate preferred first-line regimen is shown in Table 9.1.

Table 9.1: The initial and alternate regimen if the pregnant women are unable to tolerate preferred first-line regimen.

	First-line ART for	***Preferred first-line regimen***	***Alternate first-line regimen***
	HIV-positive pregnant women	Tenofovir disoproxil fumarate (TDF) + Lamivudine (3TC) + Efavirenz (EFV)	Zidovudine (AZT) + 3TC + EFV AZT + 3TC + Nevirapine (NVP) TDF + 3TC + NVP
	Name of ARV	***Dose***	***Major side effects***
1.	TDF	300 mg once daily	Nephrotoxicity, hypophosphatemia
2.	3TC	300 mg once daily	Very few side effects, hypersensitivity, rarely pancreatitis
3.	EFV	600 mg once daily	Neuropsychiatric symptoms like hallucinations, suicidal ideations, nightmares, vivid dreams, etc.
4.	Lopinavir/ Ritonavir (LPV/r)	400/100 mg twice daily [dose of FDC tablet of LPV (200 mg)/r (50 mg)—2 tablets twice daily]	Gastrointestinal disturbances, glucose intolerance, lipodystrophy and hyperlipidemia

Principles of Management

- ART should be started as early as possible and continued throughout pregnancy, delivery, breastfeeding and thereafter lifelong.
- If the patient presents very late in pregnancy even at 36 weeks of gestation, ART should be initiated immediately.

INTRAPARTUM MANAGEMENT

A decision about the mode of delivery should be made between 34 weeks and 36 weeks based on the plasma viral load, CD4 T-lymphocyte count, current maternal medical status, and ART.

Intrapartum Anti-retro Viral Therapy

Women who are on lifelong ART should continue the same medicines at the usual schedule including during labor and delivery.

Mode of Delivery

Planned vaginal delivery:

- Prenatally diagnosed patients with good maternal health, no coinfections, a plasma viral load less than 1,000 copies/mL, and on combination ART can be planned for vaginal delivery.
- In patients diagnosed during the present pregnancy, viral load levels will guide the mode of delivery. If it is less than 1,000 copies/mL with low additional risk factors, the patient can still be planned for vaginal delivery with continuation of ART during labor.
- In patients diagnosed during labor, intravenous Zidovudine and oral nevirapine should be started. Samples for viral load, CD4 counts, and resistance testing should be sent. A pediatrician should be informed.
- If patient is in early stages of labor with intact membranes, and the viral load is less than 1,000 copies/mL then she can be allowed to deliver vaginally. Cesarean section should be planned if the viral load is more than 1,000 copies/mL, after at least 2 hours of nevirapine.
- If the patient is already at an advanced stage, labor should be expedited. In all vaginal deliveries, precautions detailed in Box 9.1 here should be observed during labor.

Role of Cesarean Section

According to NACO and US Centers for Disease Control and Prevention (CDC) recommendations, a Cesarean section should be done only if there is an obstetric indication for the same.

A planned Cesarean section should be considered in patients with high viral loads, coinfection with hepatitis C and poor maternal health at 38 weeks.

Box 9.1: Precautions during labor.

- Maintain partograph
- External electronic fetal monitoring
- Avoid artificial rupture of the membranes
- Expedite labor
- Fetal blood sampling/fetal scalp electrodes are contraindicated
- Avoid instrumental delivery. However, if required, low cavity/outlet forceps delivery is preferred to a ventouse
- Bathe the baby with soap and water before any invasive procedure
- Continue ART that was being used antenatally during labor
- Start intravenous (IV) zidovudine infusion 2 mg/kg body weight over 1 hour as a loading dose, and continue the infusion at 1 mg/kg/hour till delivery
- In developing countries where IV zidovudine is not available, start with oral zidovudine one tablet 300 mg 3 hours till delivery
- Infant prophylaxis—zidovudine for 6 weeks

Box 9.2: Precautions during elective cesarean section.

- Start intravenous zidovudine/oral tablet 3 hours prior to a planned section
- Continue the previous ART regimen
- Delay rupture of the membranes till the delivery of the head of the baby through the uterine incision
- Clamp the cord early
- Ensure meticulous hemostasis
- Provide adequate antibiotic cover

Patients with negligible viral loads but not wanting a vaginal delivery can be planned for Cesarean section at 39 weeks.

Use of ARV drugs during Cesarean section:

- Women on lifelong ART should continue the same ART regimen.
- For elective Cesarean sections, ART should be started before the operation (Box 9.2).
- Pregnant women requiring an emergency Cesarean section and not on ART, should receive ART before surgery and continue thereafter.

All HIV-infected pregnant women requiring Cesarean section should receive prophylactic antibiotics. Postpartum fever is the most frequently reported complication in these patients.

SPECIAL CIRCUMSTANCES

Preterm labor and preterm rupture of the membranes:

- There is an increased risk of preterm labor in patients taking combination drug therapy initiated in the first trimester.

- Patients with threatened preterm labor should be given tocolytics, steroid cover, and injectable antibiotics.
- If the gestational age is less than 32 weeks, the infant will not initially be accepting oral feeding and hence the intrapartum drug of choice is oral nevirapine 200 mg given 2 hours prior to delivery, 600 mg of oral tenofovir and intravenous zidovudine.
- In case of premature rupture of the membranes, the risk of chorioamnionitis is high. Patients can be allowed to deliver vaginally only in the absence of genital infection, chorioamnionitis and other obstetric contraindications.
- Prolonged rupture of membranes increases the risk of transmission and neonatal morbidity.

Prolonged pregnancy beyond 41 weeks:

- Pregnancy can be induced in a low viral load scenario if the cervix is favorable. Prostaglandins are not contraindicated in HIV-infected pregnant women.

POSTPARTUM MANAGEMENT

During the postpartum period, the mother should be given social and moral support from her husband, family members as well as from society as this is a stressful period for her as she has multiple roles and responsibilities. *Mother and infant care includes the following important points*:

- HIV-positive mothers should take ART regularly.
- Daily nevirapine prophylaxis for infants for 6 weeks.
- Care and follow-up of the infant including clinic visits and immunization follow-up; early infant diagnosis (EID) and cotrimoxazole prophylactic therapy (CPT) initiation and continuation for at least 18 months.
- Regular visits to the ART centers by the mother (Flowcharts 9.1 and 9.2).
- Exclusive breastfeeding for 6 months and for 1 year in EID-negative babies and it can be extended to 2 years in EID-positive babies. Weaning foods can be initiated after 6 months of age in all babies including both breastfed as well as replacement fed babies. Pediatric ART can be considered later.
- Insertion of intrauterine device (IUD) is advisable for all HIV-infected mothers after 6 weeks of delivery if postpartum IUD (PPIUD) has not been inserted within 48 hours of delivery. Concomitant use of condoms with intrauterine contraceptive device (IUCD) will prevent unwanted pregnancies (dual protection).
- Male sterilization should be encouraged in these cases [no scalpel vasectomy (NSV) between 18 months and 2 years, once the baby's survival has been ensured].

Flowchart 9.1: Anti-retro viral therapy in babies of HIV-positive mothers.

Anti-retro viral therapy in babies of HIV-positive mothers

↓

Babies on exclusive breastfeed (EBF) for the first 6 months

Mother
Lifelong ART initiated as early as possible including entire breastfeeding period

Infants

i. At birth: NVP prophylaxis immediately after birth and up to 6 weeks
ii. At 6 weeks:
   a. After NVP prophylaxis, cotrimoxazole prophylactic therapy (CPT) should be started and continued till 18 months of age
   b. Routine immunization protocol as for normal babies should be followed
   c. Early infant diagnosis (EID): Dried blood spot (DBS) test should be done for all babies of HIV-positive mothers at 6 weeks; if positive do whole blood sample (WBS) test and if this is also positive, then pediatric ART should be initiated irrespective of CD4 count for babies less than 2 years
   d. Mixed feeding is not advisable for first 6 months, i.e. avoid other milk, fruit juices or even water with breastfeeding

Postpartum Care and Follow-up

- Every mother should be evaluated for postpartum infectious complications.
- Contraception counseling should be offered to all HIV-infected women and their partners in the postpartum period which should include barrier contraception, IUD adoption and motivation for non-scalpel vasectomy at 18 months. EID program and ART program for mother/child should be followed as indicated.

Contraception

Hormonal contraceptives: Oral hormonal contraceptives [oral contraceptive pills (OCPs): norethindrone/ethinylestradiol] are effective but prone to drug interactions most likely with:

- Non-nucleotide reverse transcriptase inhibitors, e.g. efavirenz and nevirapine
- Protease inhibitors
- Medicines for comorbidities, e.g. rifampicin.

Intramuscular depot medroxyprogesterone acetate has shown efficacy in HIV-positive women and less interaction with ART.

Flowchart 9.2: Anti-retro viral therapy in babies of HIV-positive mothers.

Anti-retro viral therapy in babies of HIV-positive mothers

↓

Babies on exclusive replacement feeds (ERF) for the first 6 months

↓

Mother
Lifelong ART initiated as early as possible though the mother is not feeding the baby

Infants

i. At birth: NVP prophylaxis immediately after birth and up to 6 weeks
ii. At 6 weeks:
   a. After NVP prophylaxis, cotrimoxazole prophylactic therapy (CPT) should be started and continue till 18 months of age, and may be thereafter, if baby is positive
   b. Routine immunization protocol as for normal babies should be followed
   c. Early infant diagnosis (EID): Dried blood spot (DBS) test should be done for all babies of HIV-positive mothers at 6 weeks; if positive do whole blood sample (WBS) test and if this is also positive, then pediatric ART should be initiated irrespective of CD4 count for babies less than 2 years
   d. Mixed feeding is not advisable for first 6 months, i.e. avoid other milk, fruit juices or even water with breastfeeding. No breastfeed is advisable for first 6 months

Source: Adapted with permission from National AIDS Control Organization (NACO). Updated Guidelines for prevention of parent to child transmission (PPTCT) of HIV using multi drug anti-retroviral regimen in India. December, 2013.

Zidovudine is not affected by these interactions with oral contraceptives or intramuscular depot medroxyprogesterone acetate.

Barrier contraceptives:

- Condoms are the most commonly used and are effective in preventing transmission but not that effective for prevention of pregnancy.
- Female condoms and diaphragms are not very popular but the risk is further reduced due to concomitant use of spermicidal jellies.

Intrauterine contraceptive devices: They provide safe and efficacious contraception in HIV-infected patients. They have been shown to be better than oral contraceptives.

Breastfeeding

Human immunodeficiency virus transmission can occur even with antepartum and postpartum ART; this has been attributed to breastfeeding. The risk of HIV infection due to breastfeeding is difficult to determine due to the mixed picture of in utero, intranatal, and early postnatal transmissions.

In resource-limited settings, the risk of infectious diseases, malnutrition, and unavailability of safe water supersedes the risk of HIV transmission. Hence,

Box 9.3: Risk factors increasing vertical transmission.

- Early months of breastfeeding
- Maternal high viral load
- Seroconversion during the perinatal period
- Maternal low CD4 counts
- Low HIV-1 specific immunoglobulins (IgA, IgM) in breast milk
- Low levels of secretory leukocyte protease inhibitor (SLPI) protein in infant saliva
- Presence of mastitis, breast abscesses, cracked nipples
- Mixed feeding

even though replacement feeding has shown a lower risk of transmission than exclusive breastfeeding in the developed world, in the developing world exclusive breastfeeding with ART-prophylaxis is the preferred choice.

Risk Factors Increasing Vertical Transmission

Risk factors increasing vertical transmission have been shown in Box 9.3.

CONCLUSION

- Prevention of HIV infection is an important concern, and to prevent vertical transmission, all pregnent women should be tested.
- Couples should be offered the option of medical termination of pregnancy (MTP), if they are not ready to take or are unable to afford ART.
- There are increased chances of first trimester pregnancy loss and the chances of ectopic pregnancy are higher with HIV infection.
- Factors affecting transmission include maternal, viral, obstetric and fetal factors.
- Perinatal HIV infection transmission can occur during the antepartum, intrapartum or postpartum periods.
- Cesarean section should be done only if there is an obstetric indication for the same.

SUGGESTED READING

1. National AIDS Control Organization (NACO). Updated Guidelines for prevention of parent to child transmission (PPTCT) of HIV using multi drug anti-retroviral regimen in India. December 2013.
2. Obstetrics and Gynecology: A Case-based Approach. Chapter 14: HIV-positive pregnancy. pp. 251-74.
3. Recommendations for use of antiretroviral drugs in pregnant HIV-1-infected women for maternal health and interventions to reduce perinatal HIV transmission in the United States. AIDSInfo. [online] Available from https://aidsinfo.nih.gov/guidelines. [Accessed October 2017].

CHAPTER

10

HIV Patients Desiring Pregnant

Atul Kakar, Shweta Mittal Gupta

INTRODUCTION

With the advent of many new anti-retro viral drugs and treatment options becoming more affordable, people living with HIV/AIDS (PLHA) now are seeking advice on whether they can extend their families. It is also important to realize that up to 80% of PLHA are in their reproductive period and these patients have a right to plan families. With the advances in scientific knowledge, the scope of reproductive medicine in HIV has also been amplified. The problems, which PLHA patients usually face, are family planning, sexually transmitted diseases, contraceptive, and sexual violence.

Recently, the WHO upgraded their recommendations of when to start anti-retro viral therapy (ART) for people living with HIV. They recommend that ART should be initiated in adults at any CD4 cell counts and in all pregnant and breastfeeding women irrespective of their CD4 cell counts.

PREGNANCY: A POSSIBILITY IN HIV-POSITIVE PATIENTS

Pregnancy is a possibility in HIV/AIDS patients. The pregnancy rate in PLHA is less than in the general population, but pregnancy outcomes are similar. If the mother has HIV/AIDS, the infants can be infected during pregnancy and the mother-to-child route (MTCT) is the most common route to get HIV in children and infants. It is estimated that each day approximately 1,000 infants acquire HIV due to MTCT during pregnancy, delivery, or breastfeeding. If the mother is on highly active anti-retro viral drugs (HAART) or also combined anti-retro viral drugs (C-ART) then the risk of transmission to baby is greatly reduced. Data now suggest that there is little effect of pregnancy on HIV progression. In a meta-analysis, it was suggested that in the presence of C-ART, pregnancy is associated with a blunted (attenuated) progression of HIV. The abortion rate is lower once the patient is on C-ART (Table 14.1).

Table 14.1: Risk of vertical transmission.	
Without ART	15–40%
With monotherapy zidovudine	8–10%
With ART	2%

(ART: Anti-retro viral therapy).

Does HIV Infection Affect Fertility?

In Males

- HIV has a detrimental effect on the semen resulting in low-sperm counts, low motility, and low volumes.
- The lower the CD4 cell counts the higher is the progression of the disease, which also affects the semen characteristics.
- HAART, itself, decreases DNA integrity in the sperm leading to DNA damage. Thus even though the viral load is reduced, sperm DNA can still be affected by HAART.

In Females

- In women with HIV, there is a decreased phagocytosis by polymorphonuclear leukocytes causing impaired cellular antigen-presenting function, which delays the onset of symptoms. The course of pelvic infections is prolonged.
- HIV infection influences ovarian reserve and immunosuppression, which can lead to early menopause. However, since the human oocyte/cumulus cells have no receptors for HIV, the virus does not impact oocyte directly.
- HAART causes direct mitochondrial dysfunction in the oocyte.

PRECONCEPTION COUNSELING

During this period, knowledge about safer sexual practices, lifestyle changes (e.g. stopping alcohol, smoking, and drugs) and contraceptive methods should be discussed.

Counseling should also include nutrition, rest, and warning signs of problems in pregnancy. The physician should also discuss planning of the birth, institutional/hospital delivery, and breastfeeding within an hour of delivery.

All HIV-positive women should plan pregnancy when the plasma viral load is below the detectable level.

Principles of fertility of management of HIV-infected patients:

- Reduce viral load in the infected partner
- Decrease the noninfected partner's exposure and infection risk
- Discuss risk reduction strategies with the couple
- Obtain informed written consent.

SAFER OPTIONS FOR HIV-POSITIVE PATIENTS TO BECOME PREGNANT

If one patient is positive and the other is HIV negative, they are called a serodiscordant couple. Flowchart 10.1 describes the options available.

Flowchart 10.1: Safer options for HIV positive patients to become pregnant.

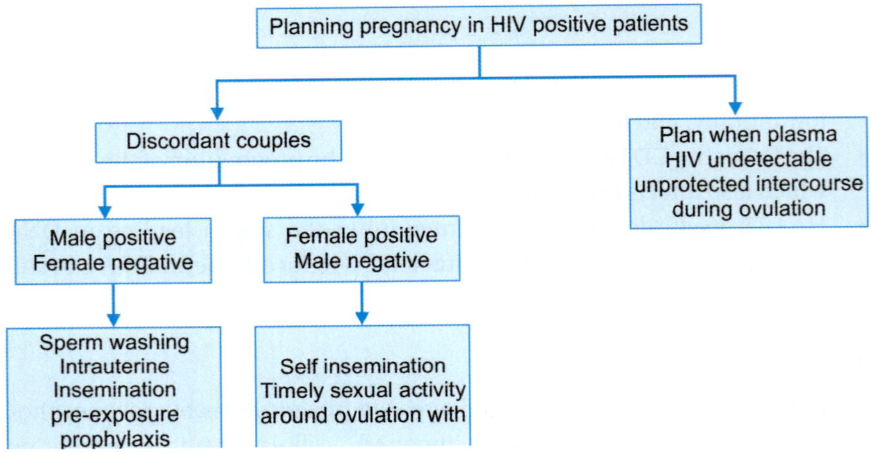

There are three major ways to reduce the transmission to the baby, i.e.:

1. *Pre-exposure prophylaxis*: A short course of HIV medication is given to the HIV-negative partner before sexual exposure (starting 30 days before and 30 days after sexual contact).
2. *Timing of sexual activity*: The partners to be engaged in sexual activity only during ovulation.
3. *Assisted reproduction*: These techniques are done by fertility clinics and include procedures like cup insemination, intrauterine insemination (IUI), and in vitro fertilization (IVF). These procedures are done after a sperm wash. For discordant couples with HIV-infected women, the safest conception method is artificial insemination or self-insemination during the periovulatory period. For discordant couples with HIV-infected men, the donor sperm from anonymous HIV-noninfected man with artificial insemination is the safest option. The sperm analysis should be done in an attempt to prevent infectious genital fluid exposure.

The clinical scenario are given below:

1. In case male is positive for HIV and female is negative.
   There are chances of infecting the partner. HIV load should be bear minimum and husband should not have any other sexually transmitted

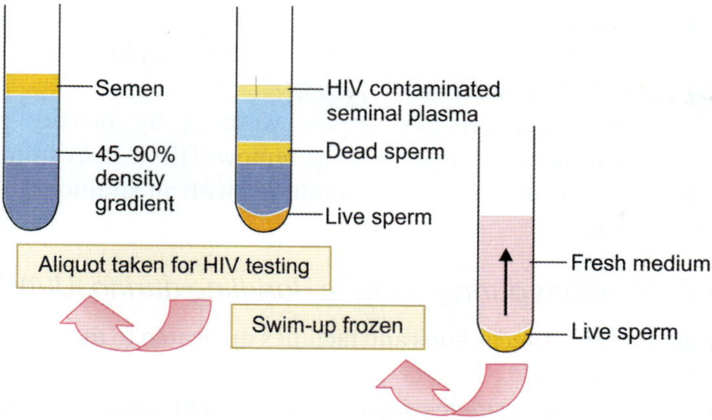

Fig. 10.1: Stages of sperm preparation.

disease. Sperm wash should be done and IUI should be considered for pregnancy. Figure 10.1 gives stages of sperm preparation.

2. *If the female is positive for HIV and the male is negative*:
   In this case, the male can plan intercourse at the time of ovulation and prior to intercourse undergoes pre-exposure prophylaxis. This can further reduce the chance of the male becoming positive. The other option is artificial insemination of the female.
3. In case both partners are positive, conception should not be considered till the viral load in undetectable. Also, there should not be any other sexually transmissible disease in the partners.

Principles of Semen Preparation (Flowchart 10.2)

Flowchart 10.2: Principles of semen preparation.

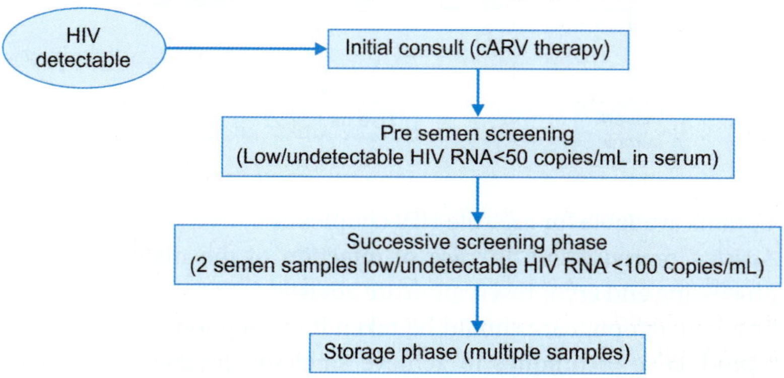

- HIV viral RNA and proviral DNA are found free in seminal plasma and in non-sperm cells
- Receptors (CD4, CCR5, CXCR4) are expressed only by non-sperm cells

- Prepared sample is tested by reverse transcription polymerase chain reaction (rt-PCR) before use and only HIV-free samples should be used for intrauterine insemination
- It has been suggested that sperm washing by density gradient centrifugation alone is insufficient to remove HIV-1 RNA from semen and that the procedure should be combined with an additional swim-up separation step.

Special Precautions during Gamete Handling during IUI/IVF

- Requires specific precautions and facilities dedicated to the processing of an infectious agent
- Potentially infected gametes and embryos must be handled separately in a special biosafety cabinet workstation
- Dedicated-use incubators and storage tanks should be devoted solely to specimens from men known to be HIV positive
- Separate laboratory
- Washing techniques of semen before storage
- Separate gamete storage tanks
- Double bagging/sealing—to prevent contact with liquid nitrogen.

Storage Phase (Multiple Samples) (Flowchart 10.3)

Flowchart 10.3: Storage phase

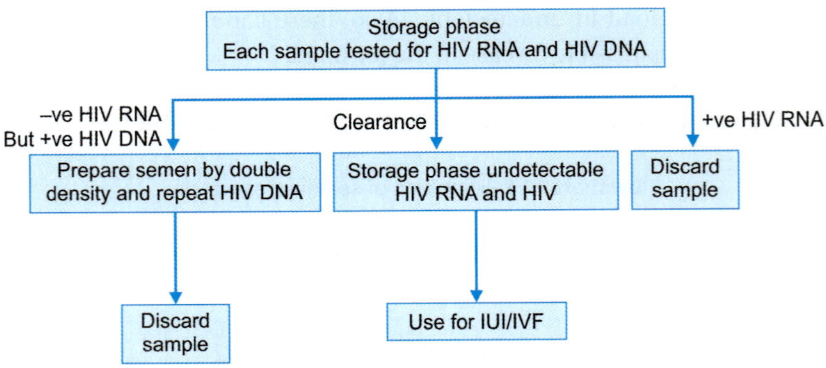

The options available for infertile HIV couples are:

- *Assisted reproduction*: In case of infection of the male partner sperm processing and cryopreservation are advised.
- Post conception, care should be taken if conception is through assisted reproductive techniques to achieve singleton pregnancy as there is a higher risk of vertical transmission of the virus in preterm labor or during premature rupture of the membranes. Although the mother should be encouraged to breastfeed, if mother is positive the choice for top feeding should be offered.

Patients should receive C-ART to decrease the risk of perinatal transmission. Drug resistance testing should be done prior to the initiation of medication. The benefit of C-ART outweighs the risk of fetal exposure to such drugs and this should be told to the patient. The drugs which are safe are:

1. Dual nucleoside reverse transcriptase inhibitors—Abacavir/Lamivudine, Tenofovir/Emtricitabine or Lamivudine or Zidovudine/Lamivudine.
2. Protease inhibitors—Ritonavir-based (Atazanavir or Darunavir or Lopinavir)
3. Non-nucleoside reverse transcriptase inhibitors—Efavirenz-based regimen should be initiated after 8 weeks of pregnancy.
4. Integrase inhibitor—Raltegavir is a new group of drugs which can also be given in pregnancy.

Recommended first-line regimen for HIV-infected pregnant women is Tenofovir (TDF) (300 mg) + Lamivudine (3TC) (300 mg) + Efavirenz (EFV) (600 mg) [if there is no prior exposure to NNRTIs (NVP/EFV) at any gestational age]. In case patient has received ART earlier then Efavirenz can be subsisted by Zidovudine, Nevirapine or Lopinavir/Ritonavir combination.

CONCLUSION

- The viral load in the blood sometimes does not correlate with levels in the semen and genital secretions.
- If the patient is on effective ART, the chances for perinatal transmission is low.
- The discordant couple should have intercourse without a condom at ovulation in case the female is positive. Intrauterine in secretion and sperm processing should be done in case of infection of the male partner.

SUGGESTED READING

1. Calvert C, Ronsmans C. Pregnancy and HIV disease progression: a systemic review and meta-analysis. Tropical Medicine & International Health. 2015;20:122-45.
2. Ford N, Lynne M, Shuber Z, et al. Safety of Efavirenz in the first trimester of pregnancy: an updated systemic review and meta analysis. AIDS. 2014;28(Suppl 2):S123-131.
3. Guidelines on when to start antiretroviral therapy and on pre-exposure prophylaxis for HIV, WHO 2015.
4. http/aidsinfo.nih.gov/guideline. Recommendations for use of antiretroviral drugs in pregnant HIV-1 infected women for maternal health and intervention to reduce perinatal HIV transmission in the United Stated. Last accessed on 24.11.2015.
5. Massad LS, Springer G, Jacobson L, et al. Pregnancy rates and predictors of conception, miscarriage and abortion in US women with HIV. AIDS. 2004;18:281-6.
6. Shetty AK. Epidemiology of HIV infection in women and children: a global perspective. Curr HIV Res. 2013;15:81-92.
7. Tsague L, Abrams EJ. Commentary: anti-retroviral treatment for pregnancy and breast feeding women—the shifting paradigm. AIDS. 2014;28(Suppl 2):S119-121.

SECTION 5

Opportunistic Infections

CHAPTER

11

Diagnosing Tuberculosis and Nontuberculous Mycobacterial Diseases

Reena Raveendran, Chand Wattal

INTRODUCTION

The World Health Organization (WHO) estimated that, in 2015, there were about 10.4 million new (incidents) cases of tuberculosis (TB) worldwide. 1.2 million (11%) of all new TB cases were among people living with the human immunodeficiency virus/acquired immunodeficiency syndrome (PLHA). An estimated 1.4 million patients died of tuberculosis in that year, and an additional 0.4 million patients died due to TB disease among those with PLHA. India accounts for approximately 26% of the world's annual incidence of TB. Every year, around 2 million new cases and 300,000 deaths are attributed to TB in India. The problem is grave in HIV-infected patients who are more susceptible to TB infection. These patients are more likely to progress to active TB disease and to develop severe forms of the disease like disseminated TB and extrapulmonary TB (EPTB). The mortality rate is also higher in HIV-TB coinfected patients. Rapid and accurate diagnosis is critical for timely initiation of antituberculous treatment. Prompt and accurate diagnosis is also the key element in any TB control program aiming at preventing further spread to contacts. With the availability of new diagnostic tools and utilization of well-planned strategies, timely diagnosis and effective treatment is possible for TB patients.

TESTING AND SCREENING STRATEGIES

Testing and Screening for Pulmonary Tuberculosis

Testing for pulmonary TB (PTB) is indicated in:

- A person with signs and symptoms suggestive of TB including cough and/or fever more than or equal to 2 weeks, significant weight loss, hemoptysis, etc.
- An abnormal chest radiograph has to be evaluated for TB.

Screening for PTB:

- Indicated in PLHA, malnourished patients, cancer patients, diabetics, immune-suppressed patients, etc.

Testing for EPTB:

- Indicated in all patients with signs and symptoms suggestive of EPTB. Appropriate specimens from suspected sites of involvement must be subjected to evaluation by microscopy, culture, nucleic acid amplification tests (NAAT), or histopathological examination.

Testing for drug-resistant TB:

- *Diagnosis of multidrug-resistant TB (MDR-TB)*:
  Testing for drug resistance should be undertaken for patients with a presumptive diagnosis of MDR-TB, in cases of failed first-line drug therapy, those with a history of close contact with MDR-TB patients (or rifampicin-resistant TB), positive sputum smear examination on follow-up during first-line drug therapy, TB patients with a previous anti-TB treatment history and proven or presumptive TB cases among PLHA. Testing for drug resistance may be carried out with the technology available, a rapid molecular drug susceptibility testing (DST) as the first choice or culture (automated liquid culture system/solid media) followed by phenotypic DST.
- DST, if available, should be offered to all diagnosed tuberculosis patients prior to the start of antituberculosis therapy (ATT).
- *Diagnosis of extensively drug-resistant TB (XDR-TB)*:
  When diagnosed as MDR-TB, or only rifampicin resistance, the patient must be advised to get his or her sputum tested for DST for second-line drugs using the WHO approved methods (phenotypic or genotypic), as per the availability.

DIAGNOSTIC TECHNOLOGY

Microscopy

Direct smear microscopy has always been the primary method for diagnosing TB in the developing countries. Smear microscopy is fast, simple, easily available, inexpensive, and is also considered specific for acid-fast bacilli (AFB) diagnosis in high-burden countries. In an effort to improve the efficiency, WHO's current policy on usage of microscopy for TB diagnosis recommends that only two specimens need to be examined in settings where good quality microscopy is being practiced with appropriate external quality assessment. A case is defined as someone with one positive smear that is at least 1 AFB when at least 100 microscopic fields are examined. In March 2010, WHO recommended that two sputum samples collected on the same day may be screened by microscopy giving results comparable to spot testing on different days. In this strategy, the patient may be started on treatment during the first visit to a healthcare facility and thereby reducing patient dropouts. The different methods of microscopy are as follows.

Light Microscopy by Ziehl-Neelsen Staining

Direct Ziehl-Neelsen (ZN) staining (Fig. 11.1) is a suitable method for use in laboratories of all levels, including peripheral healthcare facilities. It has a sensitivity of detecting 10^5 organisms/mL of the specimen. Studies have shown that processed sputum specimens do not yield any better results than a directly prepared smear from the specimen; therefore, the use of prior processing of sputum is not recommended.

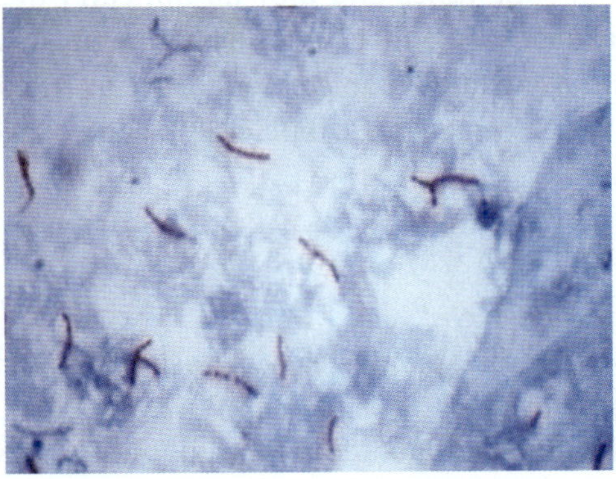

Fig. 11.1: Ziehl-Neelsen staining for mycobacteria.

Fluorescent Microscopy

The development of fluorescent dyes (e.g. auramine, rhodamine) that bind to the cell wall of mycobacteria has brought in considerable improvements in the yield of smear microscopy (Fig. 11.2) by increasing the sensitivity by ~10% compared to ZN staining. This can detect 10^{3-4} bacteria/mL of the specimen, but it is not suitable for peripheral laboratories due to its high cost, the power requirements of a mercury vapor lamp, appropriate maintenance, and storage of the fluorescent microscopes.

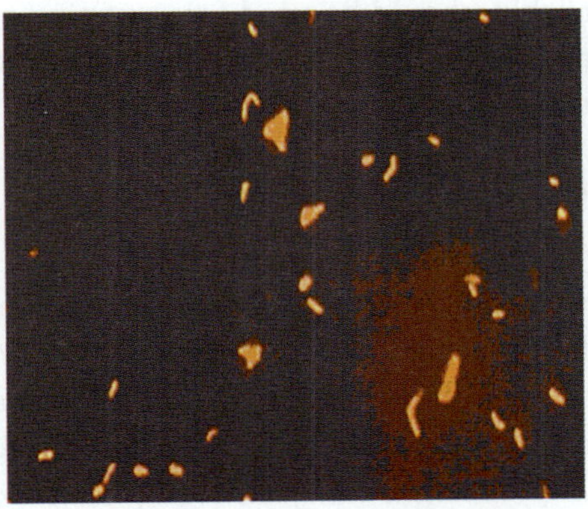

Fig. 11.2: Direct fluorescent staining for mycobacteria.

Light-emitting Diode Fluorescent Microscopy

Light-emitting diodes (LEDs) are a relatively inexpensive source for fluorescent microscopy. The power requirement is less in case of LED microscopes or LED attachments on light microscopes, than the conventional fluorescent microscopes and these systems can even work on batteries. Also, the bulb used in LED microscopes have a longer half-life compared to fluorescent microscopes using mercury vapor lamps, there is no requirement of excitation and cooling times and they do not carry the risk of potential exposure to ultraviolet (UV) light. The development of LED microscopes facilitates the use of facilities management (FM) at peripheral healthcare facilities and the WHO recommends replacing ZN and conventional FM with LED microscopy.

Benefits of Microscopy

- Simple and inexpensive
- Suitable for peripheral laboratories with basic minimum facilities as well as referral laboratories
- Can be safely done in laboratories with only a low level of safety precautions
- Can be used for treatment follow-up of patients.

Drawbacks

- Low sensitivity in patients with EPTB, pediatric cases, and in HIV patients.
- Cannot differentiate *Mycobacterium tuberculosis* (MTB) from nontuberculous mycobacteria (NTM)
- Cannot differentiate viable from nonviable bacteria
- Drug susceptibility cannot be done.

Chest X-ray

Chest X-ray, if available, should be used for screening patients presenting with signs and symptoms of TB. It is a highly sensitive tool but with a low specificity and is useful as a supportive test in diagnosis.

Culture, Species Identification, and Drug Susceptibility Testing

Culture is currently considered to be the most sensitive and specific method for the detection of mycobacterial disease (both *MTB* and *NTM*).The benefits of culture include species identification, DST, and molecular epidemiological typing. Mycobacteria may be cultured in solid or liquid media and can use all specimen types. The specimens are subjected to liquefaction, decontamination, and concentration methods before inoculation into solid or liquid media.

Results are available between 2 weeks and 8 weeks depending on the culture method used and the bacterial load present in the patient specimens. Solid media commonly used are either Lowenstein-Jensen (LJ) media (Fig. 11.3) or Middlebrook 7H10 or 7H11 agar media for culture as well as DST. The disadvantage of using solid media is the length of time required, which is approximately 18–24 days for culture and additional 28–42 days for DST. Therefore, solid culture results do not make a significant contribution toward deciding patient management. Mycobacteria grow faster in liquid media than on solid media. The WHO endorses the use of automated liquid culture systems (Fig. 11.4) for mycobacterial culture, which include Bactec960 MGIT (Becton Dickinson), BacT/ALERT (bioMerieux), and Myco ESP culture system (Trek Diagnostics). These are fully automated systems that detect the presence of mycobacterial growth, based on fluorometric or colorimetric methods, and can be used for culture of *MTB* and *NTM* species as well as DST of MTB. The average time taken for culture using automated

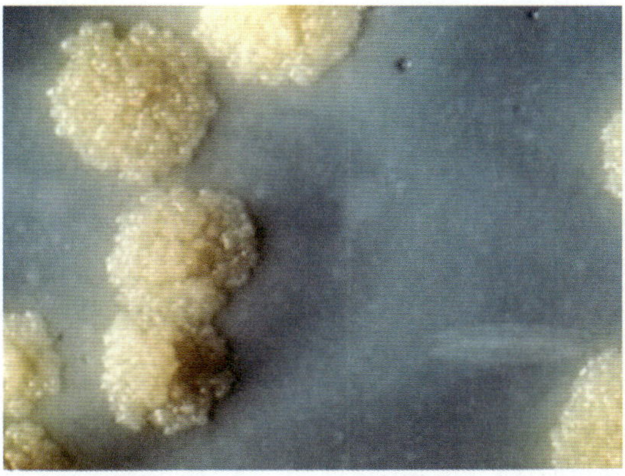

Fig. 11.3: *Mycobacterial tuberculosis* colonies on Lowenstein-Jensen (LJ) medium.

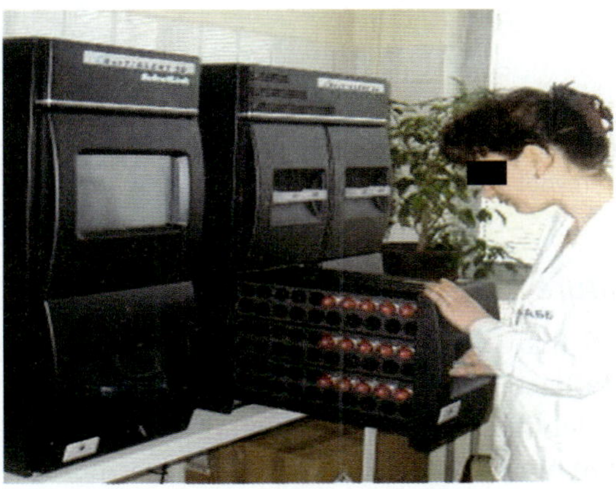

Fig. 11.4: BacT/ALERT 3D automated liquid culture system.

liquid culture systems is 10–15 days and an additional 10–14 days for DST. Mycobacterial culture, the present gold standard for diagnosing TB with 100% specificity, also has a relatively low sensitivity in clinically diagnosed cases of TB especially in EPTB. The sensitivity of culture in clinically diagnosed cases of TB varies between 82% and 93.5% in case of pulmonary TB and 25–64.6% in case of EPTB.

Once the mycobacterial growth is obtained, rapid confirmation of MTB may be done using lateral flow tests detecting *MPT64* (a specific antigen of *M. tuberculosis*). Commercially available assays include SD Ag MPT 64 rapid test (SD Bioline, Standard Diagnostics, Korea), Capilia TB Neo test (TAUNS Corporation, Japan), etc. Accuprobe test (Gen Probe, USA) is a nucleic acid-based test that detects ribosomal ribonucleic acid (rRNA) of the *MTB* complex from culture with almost 100% sensitivity and specificity. GenoType Mycobacteria CM and AS (Hain Lifesciences) are also assays used for speciation of mycobacteria from culture, which are based on polymerase chain reaction (PCR) and reverse hybridization of *23s rRNA* genes and have the capability of detecting 16 + 14 common NTM species (Fig. 11.5) in addition to the *MTB* complex.

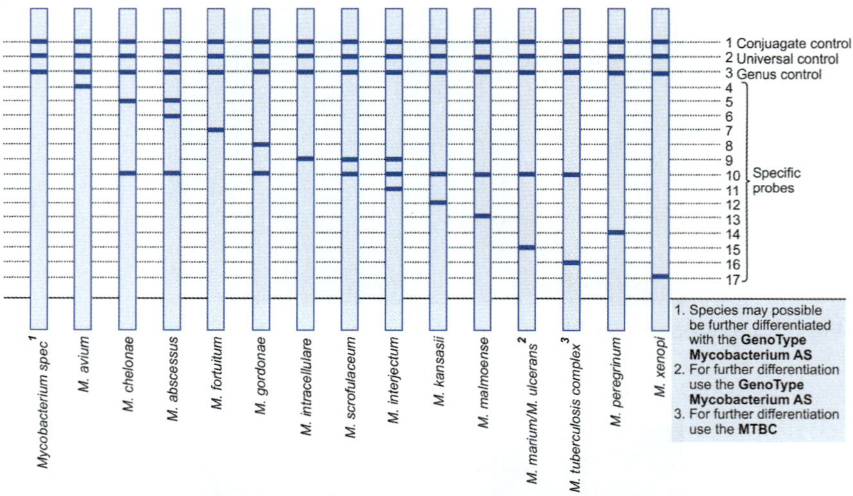

Fig. 11.5: Different nontuberculous mycobacteria species identified by GenoType mycobacteria CM (common mycobacteria) test.

Benefits of Culture

- More sensitive than microscopy. Can detect 10–100 colony-forming units (CFU) of mycobacteria
- Culture and identification provide a definite diagnosis
- Differentiation between *MTB* and *NTM* in smear-positive cases
- Can be followed by DST.

Drawbacks

- Complex and expensive
- Require biosafety and containment facilities
- Can be done only in specialized laboratories with well-trained technical staff
- Delay in the report.

Noncommercial Culture-based Methods

- MODS—microscopic observation drug susceptibility assay
- CRI—colorimetric redox indicator method
- NRA—nitrate reductase assay
- Phage-based assays
- TLA—thin layer agar assay.

Many of these methods are cheaper, giving faster results, and are more sensitive than liquid or solid culture methods. MODS, NRA, and CRI are currently approved by the WHO, for use as an interim measure in phasing out of solid culture media by automated liquid culture systems, with the condition that they are done under well-defined protocols, in reference laboratories, and follow strict quality control measures. But, none of these methods has gained popularity because of:

- Difficulties in standardization
- Need of strict QC measures
- Need for highly trained technicians
- Biosafety and containment issues
- Contamination issues.

Nucleic Acid Amplification Technologies

Nucleic acid (DNA or RNA) amplification is a sensitive method for detection of mycobacteria as well as their drug-resistance pattern and can give results faster than mycobacterial culture. Assays that are commercially available include Amplicor PCR (Roche, FDA approved), Amplified *Mycobacterium Tuberculosis* Direct (GenProbe, FDA approved), MTBDRplus (Hain Lifesciences, FDA approved, WHO endorsed), GeneXpert (Cepheid, WHO endorsed), Loop Mediated Amplification (Eiken & FIND, WHO endorsed). There are few other in vitro diagnostic (IVD)-approved NAATs (e.g. TB PCR from Qiagen, BD Probe from Becton Dickinson) with comparable performance. In addition to commercially available assays, there are many assays developed by individual centers, so-called "home brew" assays, with varying sensitivities and specificities leading to highly inconsistent results.

The sensitivity of NAATs to detect TB is as high as more than 95% in smear-positive sputum samples with high specificity, 90–100%. NAATs, in general, have a low sensitivity in smear-negative, culture-positive pulmonary specimens, and in extrapulmonary specimens. It is challenging to extract DNA from mycobacterial cells especially when the number of mycobacterial cells in the sample are few because of the peculiar physiology of the cell wall, which in turn greatly reduces the amount of DNA available for amplification. So, most of the NAATs are recommended for use only in smear-positive pulmonary specimens.

Benefits of NAAT

- TB genetic material can be detected in 2–8 hours, while culture takes weeks
- Results faster in smear-positive cases whether *MTB* complex or *NTM*
- Earlier diagnosis in smear negative cases.

NAATs fall into two broad categories:

1. Those, which detect mycobacteria directly from samples:
    - Amplified *Mycobacterium Tuberculosis* Direct Test (GenProbe)
    - Amplicor PCR (Roche).
2. Those, which detect mycobacteria along with their drug resistance.
    - *Line probe assays*: MTBDRplus (Hain Lifesciences), INNO-LIPA RIF TB (Innogenetics)
    - GeneXpert (Cepheid).

The assays, which detect drug resistance are more popular these days and both the line probe assay (LPA) and GeneXpert have been endorsed by the WHO for early detection and control of MDR-TB.

Amplified Mycobacterium Tuberculosis Direct Test

Amplified *Mycobacterium tuberculosis* direct (AMTD) uses transcription-mediated amplification (TMA) to detect 16s rRNA of *MTB* complex. The assay is FDA approved for pulmonary samples. It performs reasonably well with extrapulmonary samples, with good specificity. Has a sensitivity of 77–99% and 65–90% in pulmonary and extrapulmonary samples respectively and has a good specificity of 95–100%.

Amplicor PCR (Roche)

Amplicor PCR targets rRNA of *M. tuberculosis*. It has a sensitivity of 66–96% and 53–70% in pulmonary and extrapulmonary samples respectively and a specificity of 90–100%.

Line Probe Assay

This is a combined multiplex PCR and DNA strip reverse hybridization assay. The test screens for specific mutations encoding resistance to various drugs. Identified target regions are amplified by PCR, followed by reverse hybridization of the amplified products to a series of DNA probes immobilized on a strip. Bands appear on the strip using an enzymatic color reaction.

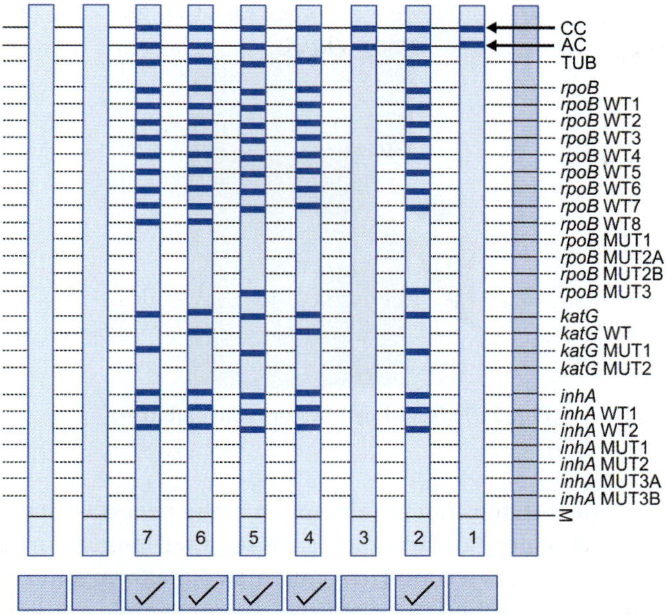

Fig. 11.6: MTBDRplus test strips.

Commercially available LPAs are:

1. *The INNO-LiPA RIF.TB*: Detects rifampicin resistance by detecting common mutations in the *rpoB* gene.
2. *The GenoType MTBDRplus assay*: Detects rifampicin resistance (by detecting common mutations in the *rpoB* gene) and isoniazid (INH) resistance (by targeting mutations in the *katG* and *inhA* genes) (Fig. 11.6).
3. *GenoType MTBDRsl*: Detects common mutations in *gyrA*, *rrs* and *embB* genes, which can lead to resistance to fluoroquinolones, aminoglycosides, and ethambutol.

MTBDRplus assay has a sensitivity of 92.5% and 98.5% for INH and rifampicin resistance detection, respectively, and a specificity of 99–100% for both. These assays are endorsed by the WHO for detection of *MTB* and simultaneous detection of drug resistance directly from smear positive pulmonary samples and culture isolates from all types of samples.

GeneXpert

The Xpert MTB/RIF test, based on the GeneXpert system (Fig. 11.7) is a cartridge-based NAAT, used for the detection of *M. tuberculosis* complex directly from patient samples by PCR amplification of mycobacterial DNA and the test also detects rifampicin resistance by detecting common mutations in the *rpoB* gene. This test has revolutionized the diagnosis of TB, by incorporating DNA extraction, amplification, and detection in a single

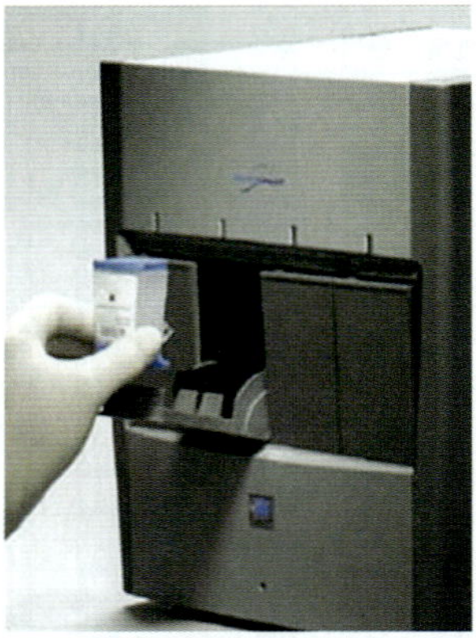

Fig. 11.7: GeneXpert system with cartridge.

cartridge. So, the test does not require much of the necessary infrastructure of a molecular laboratory and technical skills required for performing NAATs. The GeneXpert system is a completely automated platform and all the steps including extraction of the DNA from the patient sample and nested real-time PCR are carried out in the sealed cartridge, which analyzes the data, and the result is available in less than 2 hours after loading the sample. The test detects *M. tuberculosis* complex with a limit of detection of 133 CFU/mL in sputum samples. The performance is good in smear-negative sensitivity of 72.5%, culture-positive pulmonary specimens. This is a much better performance than other available PCR-based tests, which gives a good performance only in case of smear-positive pulmonary specimens. The sensitivity to detect MTB was estimated as 98–100% and 66–75% in smear-positive and -negative pulmonary samples, respectively. Sensitivity and specificity for rifampicin resistance detection is 94.4–100% and 98.3–100%, respectively. The WHO policy recommendation, 2013 on using Xpert MTB/RIF to diagnose pulmonary TB is as follows:

- Xpert MTB/RIF should be preferred over microscopy and culture, as the first diagnostic test in suspected cases of MDR-TB or HIV-associated TB.
- Xpert MTB/RIF may be preferred over microscopy and culture, as the initial diagnostic test in patients suspected of having TB.
- The recommendation is for using a single sputum specimen for diagnostic testing because of resource implications, acknowledging that processing multiple specimens increases the sensitivity of the test.
- Even when Xpert MTB/RIF is done, conventional microscopy and culture remain essential for monitoring therapy and for DST of other anti-TB agents.
- Xpert MTB/RIF detects some rifampicin-resistant strains that turns out to be susceptible by subsequent phenotypic DST-following culture. Sequencing of these strains with discordant results turns out to be

rifampicin resistant in most of the cases and those patients have a poor treatment outcome on first-line treatment.
- In case of patients, who do not have a risk for drug resistance but are detected to be rifampicin resistant by Xpert MTB/RIF, the test has to be repeated to rule out preanalytical and postanalytical errors.

The performance is reasonably good in case of extrapulmonary samples as well, and the WHO in 2013 has endorsed this assay for use in cerebrospinal fluid (CSF) and lymph node tissues and other tissue samples. But the performance is relatively poor in body fluids. There are no current recommendations for using this test in samples like stool, urine, or blood because of insufficient data regarding its utility in these specimens. Overall, the sensitivity for extrapulmonary samples has BEB estimated to be 97–100% and 47.7% respectively in smear-positive and -negative samples, respectively.

A next generation cartridge called Xpert Ultra has been developed by Cepheid with an improved sensitivity, to detect lower number of bacilli (16 CFU/mL of sputum compared to 133 CFU/mL by Xpert MTB/RIF). In March 2017, the WHO has recommended replacement of the currently used Xpert MTB/RIF cartridge with the new Xpert Ultra cartridge in all settings. Initial assessments have shown a better performance in specimens with low numbers of bacilli, like specimens from HIV-positive persons, pediatric specimens, and extrapulmonary specimens especially CSF. The accuracy of rifampicin resistance detection is also better. GeneXpert Omni is a newly developed platform, which is battery operated and portable making it suitable for use in the field.

Benefits of Xpert MTB/RIF:
- Rapid DST for rifampicin in 2 hours rather than 2–8 weeks
- No risk associated with handling of MTB cultures
- Potential for a lower cost per test compared to culture and DST.

Drawbacks:
- Cannot be used for treatment follow-up
- High cost
- Culture and DST are needed to test for resistance to other drugs
- The GeneXpert modules require annual calibration.

Loop-mediated Isothermal Amplification

Loop-mediated isothermal amplification (LAMP) is based on a temperature-independent method of DNA amplification. After the amplification step, a visual optic readout is done on an instrument that is robust and can be used even in the peripheral healthcare facilities. In August 2016, the WHO issued a recommendation for use of this test to diagnose pulmonary TB in peripheral health centers, since it requires only minimal laboratory infrastructure. When the performance of the test was compared with sputum smear microscopy

(ZN), it was observed that the TB-LAMP test detected 15% more patients among persons presenting with signs and symptoms of pulmonary TB. The test is suitable for use only in cases with a low risk of MDR-TB, since it does not detect any drug resistance.

The WHO's policy recommendations based on evaluation studies are:

- TB-LAMP may be used to replace sputum smear microscopy in adults presenting with signs and symptoms consistent with pulmonary TB.
- TB-LAMP may be used as a follow-on test to sputum smear microscopy, especially in smear-negative cases, in adults presenting with signs andsymptoms consistent with pulmonary TB.

Remarks:

- TB-LAMP should not replace the use of rapid molecular tests that detect TB and resistance to rifampicin especially among populations at risk of MDR-TB.
- There is limited evidence to suggest whether TB-LAMP has additional diagnostic value over sputum smear microscopy in PLHA presenting with signs and symptoms consistent with TB.
- These recommendations for usage of TB-LAMP are only for testing sputum specimens from patients with signs and symptoms consistent with pulmonary TB.

Biomarkers

- Adenosine deaminase (ADA) in body fluids.

Adenosine deaminase is a biomarker, which has been studied most and is in use. It is an enzyme that increases in TB because of the mycobacterial antigens leading to stimulation of T-lymphocytes.

Drawbacks

- Usage is limited only to body fluids
- Cannot differentiate TB from some other conditions that lead to an increase in lymphocytes like malignancy, rheumatoid arthritis, systemic lupus erythematosus (SLE), lymphoproliferative disorders.
- Levels may be low in HIV patients and other immunocompromised patients with low-CD4 counts.

Lysozyme in pleural fluid and tuberculostearic acid.

Their role in TB diagnosis is currently uncertain. More studies are needed in this area.

Antigen Detection Assays

The assays based on detection of lipoarabinomannan (LAM) derived from *MTB* disease are currently in use for the diagnosis of TB, but are having a poor performance. LAM, a major polysaccharide constituent of the cell wall of *MTB*, enters the bloodstream during degradation of the mycobacterial cell wall, and is filtered through the kidneys, and appears in the urine. The advantage is its potential use in diagnosis from a urine sample independent of the location of infection. It is available as ELISA as well as rapid test formats (Alere international). Its sensitivity is reasonably good (59–85%) in a high-HIV prevalent population, but is poor in a heterogeneous population with a low-HIV prevalence (13–51%). Has good specificity of 96–99%.

The 2015, the WHO recommendations on the use of LAM assays are as follows:

- LAM may be used to assist the diagnosis of TB in PLHA with suspected pulmonary or EPTB who have a CD4 cell count less than or equal to 100 cells/μL, or are seriously ill HIV-positive patients.
- Should not be used as a screening test or for diagnosis of TB in other cases.

Benefits

- Low cost
- Rapid test result
- Specimen being urine, collection is noninvasive, and easily obtainable
- Helps in diagnosing both pulmonary and EPTB.

Drawbacks

- Poor performance in non-HIV persons and in HIV-infected persons with CD4 counts more than 150 cells/μL.
- Not specific for MTB complex as other mycobacteria also produce LAM-following degradation of their cell wall.

Volatile Organic Compounds

An ever expanding field of TB diagnostic research has led us toward some new metabolic biomarkers detectable in a variety of specimens including sputum, urine or breath. When mycobacteria are active, they release volatile organic compounds (VOC). The use of VOC as a diagnostic tool has already been demonstrated to identify TB from sputum using trained Giant African pouch rats because of their acute sense of smell. Even though, pouch rats cannot be used as a global solution for improved TB diagnosis, it is observed that VOCs are a good indicator of pulmonary TB disease and are produced in a quantity sufficient to use as a diagnostic marker. A point of care device is under development to detect these metabolic biomarkers.

Benefits

- Noninvasive
- Fast.

Drawbacks

- The test is in an early stage of development
- Its role in EPTB and NTM infection is not known.

Serological Tests

Serological tests for antibody detection are not recommended for diagnosing tuberculosis and are currently banned by the WHO for use in patient diagnosis.

Tests for Detecting Latent Tuberculosis Infection

People with latent TB infection (LTBI) may develop an active disease (reactivation) in the future. The risk of TB reactivation during the entire life time of a person with LTBI is estimated to be 5–10% (as high as 60% in HIV-infected patients), with most cases developing active TB disease within 5 years after the initial infection. The tests available for detecting LTBI are:

- Mantoux test or tuberculin skin test (TST)
- Interferon gamma release assays (IGRAs).

These are indirect tests to detect TB infection by detecting memory T-cell response to *M. tuberculosis* antigens, signifying the presence of host sensitization. According to the WHO recommendations, either TST or IGRA may be used to detect LTBI in high-income countries with an estimated TB incidence less than 100 per 100,000 populations. TST should not be replaced by IGRA in low-/ middle-income countries because of the cost constraints involved.

Tuberculin Skin Test

Tuberculin skin test cannot differentiate LTBI from active TB disease. 0.1 mL of TB antigen (purified protein derivative is given as an intradermal injection into the mid-volar aspect of the forearm and examined for appearance of induration after 48–72 hours). It is recommended to use 1TU in India, as this may give a more specific report in TB endemic countries, helping us to differentiate true tuberculin sensitivity from a nonspecific reaction induced by infection with NTMs.

Drawbacks:

- Vaccination with Bacillus Calmette–Guérin (BCG) can produce a positive response.
- It has a low sensitivity in people with immunodeficiency and young children who are otherwise at the highest risk of progression to active TB.

Interferon Gamma Release Assays

The test is based on measurement of interferon-gamma (IFN-g) released by sensitized T lymphocytes of the person. The principle is that T-cells from an individual previously infected with *MTB* will release higher quantity of IFN-g, compared to naïve T-cells, when stimulated with MTB antigens. Two different commercial tests are available:

1. Quantiferon TB Gold, which uses three tuberculosis-specific antigens; the early secreted antigenic target 6 (ESAT-6), culture filtrate protein 10 (CFP 10), and the TB7.7 protein.
2. T-spot TB, which uses two tuberculosis-specific antigens ESAT-6 and CFP-10.

Benefits:

- IGRAs are more specific for LTBI compared to TST, because BCG vaccination and infection by most of the NTMs do not affect the result.
- More convenient, only a single visit of the patient required.

Drawbacks:

- Cannot separate latent infection from active TB disease.
- Children or individuals with immune-deficiency disorders can produce a false-negative or indeterminate result.
- Relatively expensive and the test needs to be performed in a laboratory.

WHO recommendations regarding the use of IGRA:

- Neither IGRAs nor TST can accurately predict the risk of an infected individual developing active TB disease.
- Neither IGRA nor TST should be used for the diagnosis of active TB disease.
- IGRAs are more costly and technically complex to perform than TST. So, replacing TST with IGRA as a public health intervention is not recommended in resource-constrained settings.

Other Recently Developed/Early Development Stage Tools

Deoxyribonucleic Acid Microarrays

Deoxyribonucleic acid microarrays are similar to LPA in principle and use oligonucleotide sequence-specific targets. A single chip accommodates hundreds of probes. So, the use of a single chip can facilitate identification of the species of mycobacteria and detection of many mutations coding for drug resistance. PCR amplification is performed first, to generate labeled DNAs, which are subsequently hybridized to various target probes immobilized on the microarray chip. After the run, the test data is developed via a scanner. Even though, commercially available automated platforms are available, they are not currently recommended by the WHO.

Unmet Needs in the Tuberculosis Diagnostics and Future Outlook

We still do not have a simple, rapid, and inexpensive point-of-care test for peripheral settings. We do not have a sensitive test for the real problem areas including smear negative, EPTB, and childhood TB. We still do not have a reliable test to detect latent TB with an increased predictive value for the development of active disease.

An algorithm including the best performing diagnostic tests currently available, for the diagnosis of *M. tuberculosis* and NTM diseases is given in Flowchart 11.1. In the present scenario, the diagnostic algorithm may be

Flowchart 11.1: Diagnostic algorithm for adult pulmonary tuberculosis.

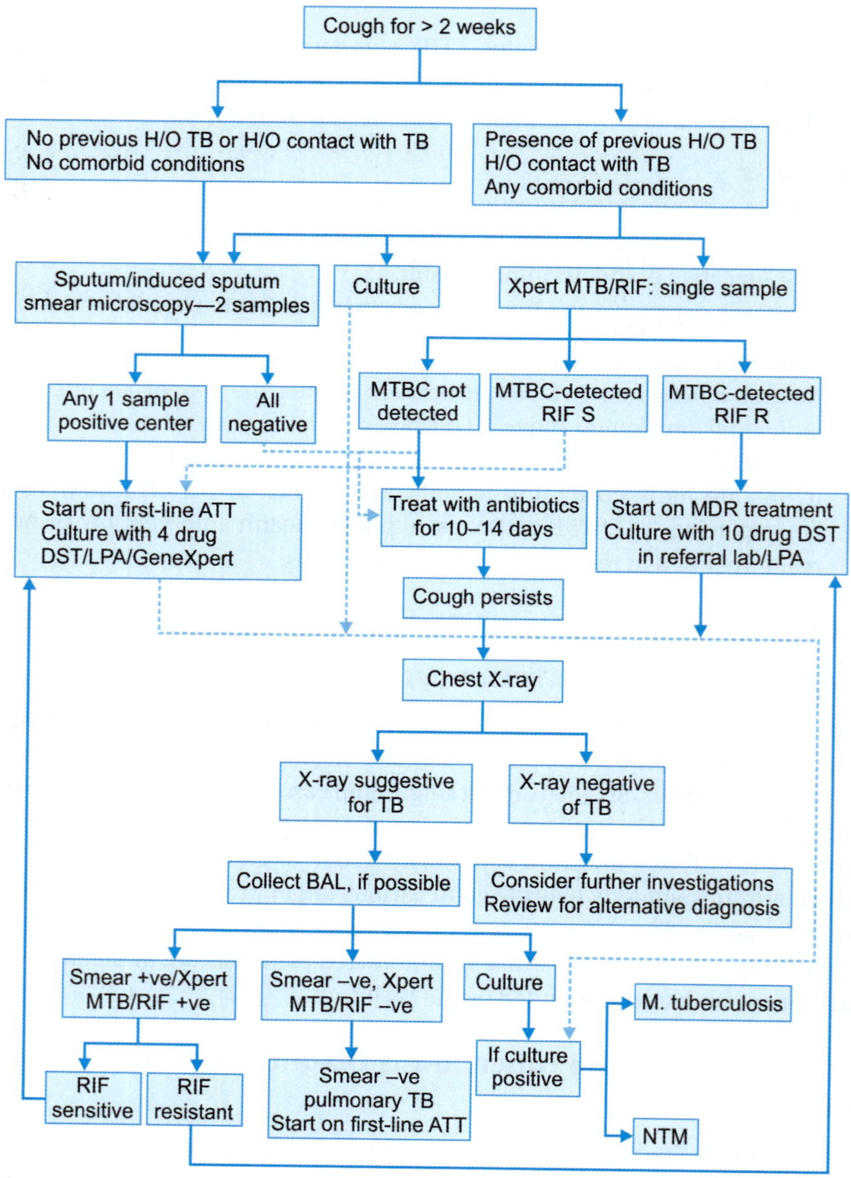

(TB: Tuberculosis; H/O: History of; MTB: *Mycobacterial tuberculosis*; MDR: Multidrug-resistant; BAL: Bronchoalveolar lavage; NTM: Nontuberculous mycobacteria).

followed by the clinicians to make optimum use of the various tests available for diagnosis of mycobacterial diseases.

CONCLUSION

- As we have seen, several diagnostic tests and strategies have already been suggested by the WHO and are being introduced into clinical use. The most important parameter is to keep a high index of suspicion by healthcare workers.
- There is also a need to improve awareness among healthcare workers by educating them and to enable them to better identify potential patients of TB.
- Healthcare workers should be encouraged to perform systematic diagnostic testing using the suggested algorithm and also to do screening in high-risk groups including PLHA and contacts of TB patients.
- Drug susceptibility testing, phenotypic or genotypic, is also very important to provide effective treatment to TB patients in the present scenario of increasing prevalence of multidrug resistance in our country.

SUGGESTED READING

1. Centers for Disease Control and Prevention. Availability of an assay for detecting Mycobacterium tuberculosis, including rifampicin-resistant strains, and consideration for its use—United States, 2013. MMWR. 2013;62:821-4.
2. Pai M, Schito M. Tuberculosis diagnostics in 2015: landscape, priorities, needs, and prospects. J Infect Dis. 2015;211:S21-8.
3. World Health Organization. (2016). Global Tuberculosis Report 2016. [online] Available from http://who.int/tb/publications/global_report/gtbr2016_executive_summary.pdf. [Accessed November 2017].
4. World Health Organization. Implementing tuberculosis diagnostics. Policy framework. Geneva: World Health Organization; 2015. WHO/HTM/TB/2015.11.
5. World Health Organization. Tuberculosis diagnostic technology landscape, 2012. Geneva: UNITAID Secretariat, World Health Organization; 2012. unitaid@who.int.
6. World Health Organization. Xpert MTB/RIF assay for the diagnosis of pulmonary and extrapulmonary TB in adults and children, Policy update. Geneva: WHO; 2013. WHO/HTM/TB/2013.16.

CHAPTER 12

Treatment of Tuberculosis in HIV

Bobby Bhalotra

INTRODUCTION

There has been a surge in the number of cases of both human immunodeficiency virus (HIV) and tuberculosis (TB) in the developing countries and this has lead to an epidemic wherein more and more patients of HIV are contacted who are suffering from TB as well. The two infections complement each other making diagnosis and treatment a major challenge. The mortality and morbidity of TB increase with the progressive decline in CD4 cell count in a HIV-positive patient; similarly, TB has a detrimental impact on HIV disease, increasing the risk of AIDS or death.

Proper and meticulous management of an HIV-infected patient with appropriate anti-retro viral therapy (ART) reduces the risk of developing TB by a significant proportion.

Diagnosis

The diagnosis of TB in HIV-infected patients is not straightforward, as due to advanced immunosuppression, these patients have atypical chest symptoms, noncavitatry pulmonary infiltrates with no particular preference for the upper lung fields. Therefore, diagnosing TB in these patients may be challenging. The laboratory tests, which may prove useful and confirmatory, include sputum analysis by acid-fast staining, rapid mycobacterial culture, GeneXpert MTB/Rif assay, and urine detection of the mycobacterial antigen. Lymph node fine-needle aspiration can be diagnostic especially in cases of mediastinal lymphadenopathy. Figure 12.1 depicts common types of tuberculosis seen in HIV/AIDS patient.

The duration of the presenting symptoms of TB prior to diagnosis is shorter in HIV-infected patients than in HIV-uninfected patients and the progression of the disease can be much faster leading to a higher mortality, hence a diagnostic tests algorithm should be rapidly followed.

Tuberculosis also causes a negative impact on the HIV disease, increasing the risk of its progression to AIDS or death. The reasons for this phenomenon are:

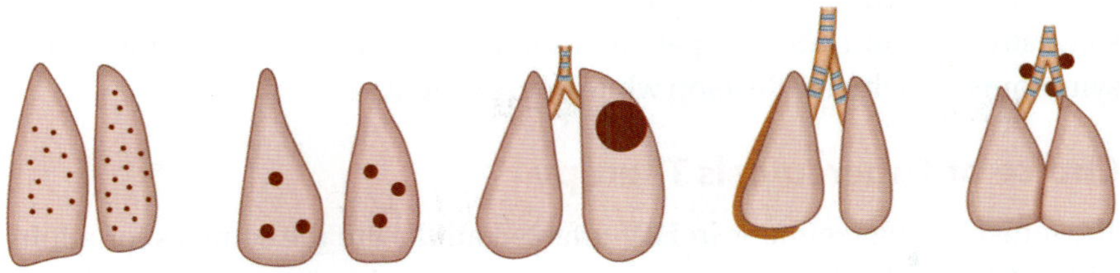

Fig. 12.1: Patterns pulmonary tuberculosis.

- Significant increases in plasma HIV viremia
- Immune reactivation, which may increase the proportion of CD4 cells which are targets for the HIV virus
- Enhanced expression of the HIV coreceptors.

IMPACT OF ANTI-RETRO VIRAL THERAPY ON TUBERCULOSIS

Effect on Tuberculosis Incidence

Anti-retro viral therapy reduces the risk of developing TB, due to improved immunity as has been shown by a higher frequency of tuberculin skin test (TST) positivity in patients on ART compared with those not taking ART.

Starting Anti-retro Viral Therapy in Tuberculosis Patients

Anti-retro viral therapy significantly reduces mortality and morbidity in patients with TB. However, the combination of ART and TB therapies can not only invite drug interactions and increase drug toxicity, but can also lead to a deterioration of TB symptoms and signs secondary to the immune reconstitution inflammatory syndrome (IRIS).

APPROACH TO THE TREATMENT OF TUBERCULOSIS IN THE HIV-INFECTED PATIENT

General Principles

- Administration of an appropriate multidrug, chemotherapeutic regimen (ATT) to combat TB
- Administration of appropriate ART for HIV
- Pay close attention to the treatment response
- Proper drug intake to be ensured
- Drug interactions should watch for and act on quickly.

A close watch has to be kept for the development of any new symptoms suggestive of the IRIS. The patient should be counseled about these new symptoms, which may develop while on treatment.

Choice of Tuberculosis Therapy

The anti-TB drug regimens in HIV-infected adults are the same as for adults without HIV infection. However, intermittent dosing is not recommended for HIV-infected patients, with CD4+ lymphocytes less than 100 lymphocytes/mm^3.

Empiric Therapy

The initial treatment for TB should include Isoniazid (INH), a Rifampicin (e.g. Rifampin or Rifabutin), Pyrazinamide, and Ethambutol for 2 months followed by Isoniazid and a Rifampicin for an additional 4 months. Pending drug-resistance testing results, medicines need to be revised if drug resistance is noted.

The initial 2-month induction phase should be administered either:

- 7 days per week (i.e. 56 doses) or
- 5 days per week (i.e. 40 doses) by directly observed therapy (DOT).

In the 4-month continuation phase of treatment, INH plus a Rifampicin should be administered daily (5–7 days) or thrice weekly.

Isoniazid: To decrease the risk of peripheral neuropathy, HIV-infected patients taking INH should also take pyridoxine supplementation. The recommended dose is 50 mg/day. Caution has to be taken as peripheral neuropathy can also be caused by certain anti-retro viral medications being used for the treatment of HIV.

Rifampicin: A rifampicin is used as a first-line drug and is a key component of TB treatment. The regimens without its use are less effective. Both Rifampin and Rifabutin are equally efficacious against *Mycobacterium tuberculosis*. The choice of drugs to be used is dependent on the ART drug interactions and their cost.

Choice of Anti-retro viral Therapy

A thorough knowledge of HIV clinical management and treatment is a prerequisite for clinicians taking care of HIV-infected patients with tuberculosis.

Anti-retro viral therapy regimens are described as having a "backbone" and a "base".

- The backbone typically consists of two nucleoside analogs.
- The base includes either a non-nucleoside reverse transcriptase inhibitor, a protease inhibitor (PI), or an integrase strand transfer inhibitor.

Efficacy of Tuberculosis Treatment

Treatment for susceptible TB is as effective in HIV-infected patients, as it is in HIV-uninfected patients, as seen by parameters such as culture conversion and completion of therapy.

Mortality rates are found to be significantly higher in HIV patients with TB than TB patients without HIV.

MONITORING THE HIV-INFECTED PATIENT ON ANTITUBERCULOUS MEDICATIONS

Directly Observed Therapy

Directly observed therapy is recommended by most TB experts and the World Health Organization (WHO) for all TB patients.

Although DOT programs are very effective in decreasing rates of primary and acquired drug resistance in developing countries where TB and HIV are endemic, DOT is associated with lower TB relapse rates and a higher percentage of patients who complete their full duration of TB therapy.

Response to Therapy

Clinical Response

Timely diagnosis and appropriate therapy have been seen to show a good response in patients with HIV infection and TB. Fever usually takes 1 month to settle and the chest radiograph shows improvement in 2–3 months.

Bacteriological Efficacy

Sputum examination is must and is required to monitor the efficacy of treatment in the HIV-infected TB patient. It should be done every fortnight in patients with positive acid-fast bacilli (AFB) smears until a negative smear is documented. This makes sure that the treatment is effective.

On the other hand, in patients with smear-negative disease, a monthly collection and examination of samples will suffice.

On completion of therapy, despite the conversion of sputum culture to negative, at least one further sputum examination should be done to confirm that the patient has indeed remained culture negative.

Clinical Deterioration

This subset of patients with both HIV and TB infection is at very high risk usually because of poor adherence to medication, inadequate drug absorption, emergence of drug resistance, onset of an opportunistic infection, or the IRIS.

Predictors of Relapse

One can predict the onset of relapse in these patients by:

- A low CD4+ lymphocyte count. This is the key risk factor for relapse in HIV-infected persons
- A cavitatry lesion on chest radiograph
- Positive sputum culture after 2 months of treatment.

If the sputum culture continues to be positive despite of 2 months of intensive antitubercular treatment, drug resistance should be suspected and the sputum should be recultured to look for possible drug resistance.

Recurrence

Recurrence of TB is more common in HIV-infected patients (24%) than in non-HIV patients (4%).

Immune Reconstitution Inflammatory Syndrome

Immune reconstitution inflammatory syndrome usually occurs in HIV patients who were recently initiated to TB medications and ART. The incidence ranges from 8% to 43%. These patients show transient clinical and/or radiographic worsening despite appropriate medication. This phenomenon happens due to a transient increase in the inflammatory response of the host due to a partial improvement of the immune response.

The risk is increased in patients who show a sudden increase in CD4 cell counts or a significant fall in viral load. Clinical manifestations in the HIV-infected patient with TB can include new or expanding lymph nodes, enlarging intracranial tuberculomas, persistent pyrexia, worsening pulmonary infiltrates, and new serositis.

Paradoxical responses are self-limited and the addition of nonsteroidal anti-inflammatory drugs or a short course of corticosteroids has been recommended, if it causes significant symptoms. However, antitubercular drugs and ART should continue unchanged. It is essential to thoroughly reevaluate the diagnosis to exclude TB mimics like lymphoma, TB treatment failure, or drug-resistant TB.

Drug-related Side Effects

Side effects due to ATT and ART are mainly hepatic and neurological. The rate of complications is higher when the therapies for the two diseases are used together than the individual use of ATT or ART. The most common side effects are rashes and hepatitis implicated to Rifampicin. Its incidence is 24% in patients with HIV and TB in contrast to 4% in patients with only TB.

Hepatotoxicity

The risk of hepatotoxicity is increased in the setting of alcoholism and chronic liver disease (e.g. hepatitis B or C virus infection), which are common comorbidities in HIV-infected patients.

To detect early drug-induced liver injury, serial monitoring with liver function tests is advised, more so in patients with possible pre-existing liver impairment.

Peripheral Neuropathy

Most commonly seen with INH.

Visual Abnormalities

Drugs like Ethambutol and Rifabutin are most common culprits in causing drug-induced visual impairment. These visual abnormalities must be differentiated from infectious diseases such as cytomegalovirus (CMV) retinitis, which is treated by antiviral medicines. If the diagnosis is not made early, untreated CMV retinitis can lead to permanent blindness.

Ethambutol causes optic neuropathy in certain patients and appearance of floaters or decrease in visual acuity may be a manifestation of Rifabutin toxicity.

Duration of Therapy

Standard Duration

- *For HIV-infected patients on ART*: For drug-susceptible TB, 2-month intensive phase of INH, a Rifampicin (e.g. Rifampin or Rifabutin), Pyrazinamide, and Ethambutol followed by a 4-month continuation of Isoniazid and a Rifampicin.
- *For HIV-infected patients not on ART*: The continuation phase is extended for an additional 3 months with a total of 9 months of therapy. The inclusion of Rifampicin in the antitubercular therapy regimens for 9 months has been noted to have lower relapse rates.

It is important to note that daily therapy is associated with lower rates of treatment failure and relapse.

When to Prolong Therapy?

The duration of TB therapy is increased in specific clinical situations like:

- Patients with cavitary disease
- Positive sputum cultures even after 2 months of intensive phase treatment, regardless of HIV status.

The duration of treatment is extended by 3 months with continuation of INH and Rifampin for a total of nine months. Treatment for 9–12 months is also recommended for patients with bone, joint, or central nervous system (CNS) TB. In case of extrapulmonary disease, the recommended treatment is for 6 months.

Adjuvant Corticosteroids

Steroids are recommended in patients with:

- CNS or pericardial disease, as they have been shown to improve the outcome.

PROGNOSIS

Clinical Outcomes

Clinical response is good for patients who have drug-sensitive TB and are regular with their treatment. Delay in diagnosis and treatment can lead to deaths, which commonly occur in the 1st month after therapy is initiated.

Impact of Anti-retro Viral Therapy on Mortality

Anti-retro viral therapy and treatment of TB should be done concomitantly. This policy is associated with a lower mortality and morbidity.

Impact of Cotrimoxazole Prophylaxis on Mortality

There is a high incidence of opportunistic infection among HIV. These infections include salmonellosis, toxoplasmosis, and bacterial pneumonia. Cotrimoxazole prophylaxis significantly decreases morbidity and mortality among patients suffering from HIV. A 46% reduction in risk of death and a 43% reduction in risk of hospitalization were seen in HIV with TB patients taking cotrimoxazole in prophylactic dose.

Drug Interactions

Drug interactions are common and important to understand when treating TB in HIV-positive patients on ART.

- Efavirenz-based ART is the preferred over non-nucleoside reverse-transcriptase inhibitor (NNRTI)-containing regimen.
- *Nevirapine-containing ART*: Virologically suppressed patients on Nevirapine-containing ART who develop TB may continue the same ART regimen. However, initiation of Nevirapine-containing ART should be avoided in patients who are already taking TB medications due to the risk of virological failure. The 2-week lead-in phase of once-daily dosing of Nevirapine is no longer recommended because it may increase the risk of virological failure.

In the patient with drug resistance or intolerance to NNRTIs, treatment options are very limited. If only Rifampin-based TB therapy is available, the only option is to use a triple nucleoside analog combination for HIV infection, although an HIV-treatment regimen composed of three nucleoside analogs is less effective than regimens using at least two classes of drugs.

Rifabutin can be used with nucleoside analogs, PIs, and NNRTIs, including Nevirapine. However, the dose of Rifabutin must be adjusted depending on the coadministered drug. Rifabutin is more expensive than Rifampin and is generally not available in resource-limited settings.

OPTIMAL TIMING OF INTEGRATED HIV AND TUBERCULOSIS THERAPY

It depends on the level of immunosuppression as measured by the CD4 count. Among patients with less than 50 cells/mm^3, early ART (within 2 weeks after initiation of TB therapy) is associated with a decreased risk of AIDS-related illness or death compared with later ART (8–12 weeks after initiation of TB therapy).

- In HIV-infected adults with CD4 cell count less than 50 cells/mm^3, initiation of ART within 2 weeks of starting TB treatment is recommended.
- In HIV-infected adults with CD4 cell count more than or equal to 50 cells/mm^3, initiation of ART within 8–12 weeks of starting TB treatment is recommended.

The timing of ART in the HIV-infected patient with TB meningitis may differ from the patient with pulmonary TB.

Tuberculosis therapy should be initiated as soon as possible in the patient who is already taking ART. If the patient has attained viral suppression and tolerates his current ART regimen, it is preferable to administer a rifampicin that will not lead to significant drug interactions that could interfere with HIV suppression.

CONCLUSION

- Therapy for pulmonary tuberculosis (TB) in HIV-infected adults must address potential drug interactions and adverse drug reactions.
- Patients with an established diagnosis of TB disease warrant prompt initiation of antituberculous therapy.
- The optimal timing depends on the patient's immune status for HIV infected patients with pulmonary TB and CD4 cell count <50 cells/microL. It is recommended initiation of ART within two weeks after starting TB treatment.
- For HIV-infected patients with pulmonary TB and CD4 count > 50 cells/microL, the recommendation are to initiation of ART within eight weeks after starting TB treatment.

- For HIV-infected patients with TB involving the central nervous system (CNS), ART should be delayed for the first eight weeks of antituberculous therapy, regardless of CD4 count.
- Patients with HIV infection who are already on ART should continue the ART regimen and initiate antituberculous therapy as soon as possible.
- Pending drug susceptibility results, an empiric four-drug regimen should be initiated (Isoniazid, Rifamycin, Rifampin or Rifabutin, Pyrazinamide and Ethambutol). The main consideration consists of selecting a Rifamycin that will minimize the likelihood of drug interactions with ART and interference with HIV viral suppression.
- When feasible, it is preferable to select an ART regimen that is compatible with a Rifampin-based antituberculous regimen. However, there are a number of drug interactions between Rifampin and anti-retro viral agents. Rifabutin is as effective as Rifampin for treatment of TB when used in combination therapy and is associated with fewer drug interactions with anti-retro viral agents than Rifampin. However, Rifabutin is more expensive than Rifampin, and distribution is limited in resource limited settings.
- For patients with TB and HIV who are receiving a Rifampin-based antituberculous regimen, we suggest an ART regimen consisting of the non-nucleoside reverse transcriptase inhibitor (NNRTI) Efavirenz, together with two nucleoside analogs.
- For patients with TB and HIV, who are receiving a Rifabutin-based antituberculous regimen, we suggest either a protease inhibitor, NNRTI or integrase inhibitor, together with two nucleoside analogs.

SUGGESTED READING

1. http://aidsinfo.nih.gov/contentfiles/guideines/Adultand AdolescentGL.pdf. Pannel on Antiretroviral Guidelines for Adults and Adolescents. Guidelines for the use of antiretroviral agents in HIV-1-infected adults and adolescents. Department of Health and Human Services.
2. http://apps.who.int/iris/bitstream/10665/255052/1/9789241550000-eng.pdf?ua=1. New: World Health Organization. Guidelines for treatment of durg-susceptible tuberculosis and patient care. Last updated on 02.01.2018.
3. http://apps.who.int/iris/bitstream/10665/255052/1/9789241550000-eng.pdf?ua=1. World Health Organization. Guidelines for treatment of drug-susceptible tuberculosis and patient care. Last updated on 02.01.2018.
4. Nahid P, Dorman SE, Alipanah N, et al. Official American Thoracic Society/centers for disease control and prevention/infectious diseases society of America clinical practice guidelines: treatment of drug-susceptible tuberculosis. Clinical Infectious Diseases. 2016;63(7):e147-95.

CHAPTER 13

Cryptococcal Meningitis—Diagnosis

Jaswinder Kaur Oberoi, Isra Halim

INTRODUCTION

The history of the *Cryptococcus* dates back to the 19th century when San Felice discovered this fungus in peach juice. Simultaneously, Busse and Buschke isolated it from the tibial lesion of a patient. The word *Cryptococcus* is derived from the Greek words *kryptos* (hidden) and *kokkos* (berry). Many of the early case reports were related to patients with cancer. From isolated case reports to an incidence of a million cases per year against the background of the human immunodeficiency virus (HIV) epidemic and the addition of other vulnerable populations, the *Cryptococcus* has achieved a special place in clinical mycology as the "sugar-coated" (because of its polysaccharide capsule) yeast that can cause life-threatening disease. It has established itself as the leading cause of adult meningitis in many parts of the world especially in sub-Saharan Africa. In Southeast Africa between 30% and 60% of adult meningitis cases have been reported, in various studies, to be cryptococcal in origin. Cryptococcal meningitis (CM) is a life-threatening disease with a high mortality (in hospital acute mortality ranging between 30% and 50% despite antifungal therapy) and high morbidity with irreversible blindness or reversible neurocognitive effects. Though the incidence of CM has decreased over the years in developed countries due to high Anti retroviral therapy (ART) coverage in HIV patients, it still remains a huge problem in Asian and African countries where widespread ART is still unavailable.

THE PATHOGEN

Taxonomy

The *Cryptococcus* is an encapsulated basidiomycete yeast of between 5 microns and 10 microns with a prominent polysaccharide capsule measuring between 1 micron to 30 microns. Budding forms, both single and multiple, are often encountered. The genus comprises over 30 species, loosely characterized as a variety of encapsulated yeasts. Though there have been occasional reports implicating other *Cryptococcus* species like *C. albidus* and

Table 13.1: ECG changes at presentation in STEMI.

Species	*Varieties*	*Serotypes*	*Molecular types*
C. neoformans	*C. neoformans var. grubii*	A	VNI, VNII
	C. neoformans var. grubii	D	VNIV
	Unclassified	AD	VNIII
C. gatti	-	B, C	VGI, VGII, VGIII, VGIV

C. laurentii in human infections, *C. neoformans* and *C. gattii* are recognized to be the major pathogenic species.

Historically, *C. neoformans* was grouped into two varieties: *Cryptococcus neoformans var. neoformans* and *Cryptococcus neoformans var. gatti.* Using rabbit polyclonal sera, five capsular serotypes of *C. neoformans* have been defined as serotypes A through D and serotype AD. Serotype A has been reallocated to a separate variety, *C. neoformans var. grubii,* serotype D is to remain in *C. neoformans var. neoformans* and the status of serotype AD strains has not been proposed. Isolates of *C. neoformans var. gatti* are serotypes B and C. *C. neoformans var. gatti* has now been reclassified into a separate species as *C. gatti. Cryptococcus* has further been classified into eight molecular types (Table 13.1). Recently, based on molecular studies, the following taxonomy changes have been proposed: *C. neoformans var. grubii* (serotype A) with three genotypes (VNI, VNII, VNB); *C. neoformans var. neoformans* (serotype D or VNIV); and five other cryptic species, *C. gattii, C. bacillisporus, C. deuterogattii, C. tetragattii,* and *C. decagattii* (serotypes B/C or VGI-IV).

Cryptococcus neoformans is the most common species isolated in immunocompromised patients and can also cause infection in apparently immunocompetent hosts. *C. gattii,* conversely, has historically been regarded as a pathogen of apparently immunocompetent patients. However, preexisting conditions and immunocompromised states have also been reported to be risk factors for infection with this species. *C. neoformans var. grubii* (Serotype A) is found worldwide and is responsible for causing approximately 95% of the cryptococcal infections. *C. neoformans var. neoformans* (Serotype D) is found in the European region and *C. gatti* has historically been restricted to tropical and subtropical regions, most recently this has been also identified in a temperate climate such as in Vancouver Island in Canada. *C. neoformans* is enriched by nitrogenous compounds present in bird guano and is typically associated with environments teeming with pigeon droppings, such as nesting areas. Yeast cells, being small in size, are easily aerosolized and inhaled. Birds, however, do not contract the disease themselves owing to their high body temperatures which are inhibitory to the yeast. On the other hand, ecological niches with flowering Eucalyptus trees (*Eucalyptus camaldulensis*) have been known to harbor *C. gatti.*

Virulence Factors

The following have been associated among several mechanisms linked to the virulence of *Cryptococcus* in animal models and humans:

- Production of enzyme: Phenol oxidase and melanin
- Growth at 37°C
- Presence of capsular polysaccharide
- Alpha Mating types
- Secreted proteinases
- Phospholipase production
- Urease production.

The key to initiate an infection by a microorganism is its ability to survive at normal body temperatures. *C. neoformans* and *C. gatti* are thermotolerant, thriving well at 37°C, thus contributing to mammalian pathogenicity. The capsule of *Cryptococcus*, one of the cardinal factors associated with virulence, is a complex polysaccharide—glucuronoxylomannan. Besides being antiphagocytic, it is responsible for many pathobiological functions establishing infection, and is a potent activator of the alternate complement pathway.

Another crucial virulence factor is the ability of *C. neoformans* to produce an enzyme phenol oxidase that converts diphenolic compounds including catecholamines into melanin. These pigments when expressed protect the yeast from oxidative host defenses. This may, in part, contribute to the relative neurotropism of *C. neoformans* as neuronal tissues rich in catecholamines are excellent substrates for phenol oxidases.

Factors contributing to neurotropism include:

- Selective evasion of host defenses
- Abundance of catecholamines
- Specific receptors for attachment of *C. neoformans* exclusive to neuronal cells
- Active macrophage phagosomal extrusion and possible escape strategy "Trojan horse model".

HOST FACTORS

Although cryptococcosis had been well recognized for over a century, the 1980s witnessed a dramatic surge in the number of cases. This corresponded with the increasing number of cases diagnosed with HIV. Cryptococcal infections soon became a common cause of morbidity and mortality among HIV-positive patients. Detailed analyses of risk factors for cryptococcosis substantiated the claim that HIV was a major risk factor associated with its development. The USA alone saw a 1500% rise in the number of cases of CM between 1981 and 1990—a period when the world witnessed the AIDS epidemic.

Table 13.2: Risk factors associated with *Cryptococcus* infections.
▪ HIV infection
▪ Immunosuppressive therapy and corticosteroids
▪ Solid organ transplant
▪ Malignancy
▪ Lymphoproliferative disorders
▪ Rheumatologic disorder
▪ Sarcoidosis
▪ Treatment with monoclonal antibody
▪ Chronic liver and renal disease
▪ Anti-granulocyte-macrophage colony-stimulating factor antibodies

Cryptococcal meningitis is frequently seen with waning cell-mediated immunity (CMI) and is an AIDS-related opportunistic infection when the CD4+ T-lymphocyte count decreases to less than 100 cells/µL. The widespread administration of highly active anti-retro viral therapy (HAART) in developed nations has resulted in a significant decline in the incidence of cryptococcosis.

Other populations at risk include patients with malignant and lymphoproliferative disorders, solid organ transplantation, treatment with corticosteroid and/or immunosuppressive therapy or monoclonal antibodies, rheumatologic diseases, autoimmune disorders such as systemic lupus erythematosus, chronic liver diseases, and renal failure (Table 13.2).

PATHOGENESIS

The primary route of infection in cryptococcosis is the inhalation of tiny infectious propagules in the environment which tend to lodge in the pulmonary alveoli. The pathogenesis of cryptococcal infection depends upon:

- Host defenses
- Virulence of the strain
- Size of the inoculum.

Although *Cryptococcus* is ubiquitously present in the environment, the prevalence of symptomatic cryptococcosis is relatively low. Thus, the incidence of exposure far exceeds the incidence of disease. This points to the fact that apparently immunocompetent hosts resist the infection and the disease sets in only when host defenses are compromised. A decline in CMI correlates with increased susceptibility to *Cryptococcus* as is seen in patients with AIDS and cellular immunodeficiencies. Literature suggests that CD4+ T cells are of paramount importance for controlling the host response to *Cryptococcus* and may protect the host from dissemination of the disease. Healthy hosts may rarely develop the disease following exposure with an unusually large inocula.

CLINICAL MANIFESTATIONS

Cryptococcus can essentially affect any organ system:

- Pulmonary
- Central nervous system
- Skin
- Prostate
- Eye

The most common sites affected are the lung and the CNS. CNS infections can present as acute, subacute or chronic meningitis, cryptococcomas of brain, spinal cord granuloma, and chronic dementia (from hydrocephalus). Most of the patients with CM present with signs and symptoms of subacute meningitis including:

- Headache present in above 75% of patients. Severe unbearable headache, either acute or subacute, without fever is a characteristic feature of CM. Headache may be due to meningeal involvement, raised intracranial tension or sinus-venous thrombosis. Headache may be accompanied by vomiting. Presence of headache has a good prognosis, probably because these patients present early in the course of the disease and hence can be diagnosed early
- Fever may be present in 65–75% cases
- Altered sensorium may be seen in 20% patients and signals a poor prognosis
- Seizures in about 8% cases.
- Ocular symptoms including visual loss due to papilledema
- Neurological examination is usually normal, neck stiffness may be present in 30% cases
- Focal neurological deficits (uncommon) may occur in immunocompetent patients due to presence of cryptococcomas
- Cranial neuropathies, especially involving the lower cranial nerves may occur in few cases due to basal arachnoiditis or due to hydrocephalus
- Cutaneous lesions are seen usually in HIV patients, including molluscum contagiosum-like lesions, acneiform lesions, purpura, vesicles, nodules, ulcers, draining sinuses, cellulitis, etc.

The clinical presentation may be markedly different in immunocompromised hosts as compared to apparently healthy hosts in which mere asymptomatic colonization may rarely be documented.

Cryptococcal meningitis in AIDS is characterized by:

- Higher burden of yeasts
- More sites of extraneural dissemination
- Possibility of a second CNS infection, such as *Toxoplasma gondii*
- Paucity of inflammatory response
- Higher incidence of clinical disease
- Higher incidence of relapse
- ART use in AIDS may lead to Immune Reconstitution Syndrome (IRIS) in cryptococcal infection.

Table 13.3: Percentage positivity of diagnostic tests in cryptococcal meningitis.

Test	*HIV-positive patients*	*HIV-negative patients*
Positive India Ink (%)	80	50
Positive CSF culture (%)	94	82
Positive blood culture (%)	47	27
Positive CSF antigen (%)	92	96
Positive serum antigen (%)	96	86

(CSF: Cerebrospinal fluid).

LABORATORY DIAGNOSIS

A lumbar puncture with manometry is imperative for diagnosing CM. A patient with suspected CM should also be examined all over the body for the presence of any subcutaneous swellings, which can also be subjected to smear and culture examination. The positivity of different laboratory tests in CM is more in patients with HIV than those without HIV (Table 13.3).

CSF Examination

- Opening pressures may be elevated more than 20 cm cerebrospinal fluid (CSF), most commonly seen in HIV patients.
- Lymphocytic pleocytosis with elevated protein and low sugar levels.

Appropriate clinical specimens depending upon the site of involvement, e.g. CSF, blood, aspirates from cutaneous lesions, respiratory specimens, etc., are subjected to the following investigations:

- Direct microscopic examination
- Culture
- Serology
- Molecular methods.

Direct Microscopy: CSF Analysis usually Reveals

- *India Ink preparation*: Specimens should be examined in an India Ink preparation for the presence of yeast cells with prominent negatively stained capsules with or without budding. When present, the buds are attached to the mother cell via a narrow base. India Ink continues to be the method of choice for CSF specimens with a sensitivity of approximately 50% in non-HIV patients and increases to 80% in patients with AIDS. Although readily available, the use of the India Ink as sole means of diagnosis is not advisable because it is relatively insensitive for low fungal burdens and also expertise is needed to distinguishing yeast cells from other inflammatory cells present in CSF samples (Fig. 13.1).

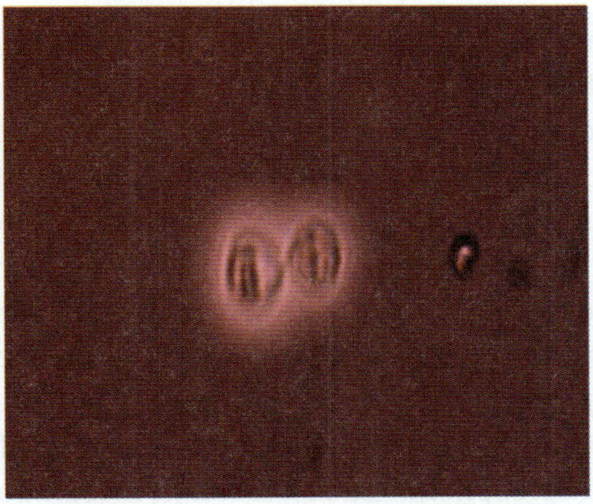

Fig. 13.1: India Ink Mount showing encapsulated budding yeast cell suggestive of *Cryptococcus* (40X).

- *Gram stain*: It usually reveals Gram-positive yeasts with narrow-based budding (Fig. 13.2).

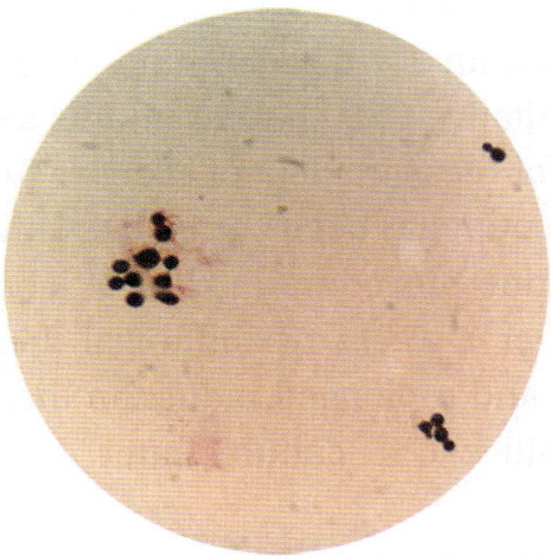

Fig. 13.2: Gram stain of cerebrospinal fluid showing Gram-positive round budding yeast cells (100X).

- *Calcofluor White (CFW) stain*: Aspirates and other specimens may be stained with a fluorescent stain, CFW, which binds to fungal chitin and examined under a fluorescent microscope. However, CFW lacks the specificity of India Ink staining.
- *Histopathology stains*: The capsular polysaccharide stains poorly in tissue sections and appears as an empty space surrounding the yeast cells. Capsule can be enhanced by the use of special stains such as Meyer's mucicarmine, periodic acid Schiff, and Alcian blue stains. As the organism produces melanin, it can be stained with Mason-Fontana stain. The organism can also be identified with Gomori methenamine silver (GMS) fungal stain as narrow-based budding yeast in tissue.

Culture

Cerebrospinal fluid culture is more than 90% sensitive and is considered the gold standard for diagnosis of CM. Cultures can also produce negative results when the fungal burden is low, though diagnostic yield can be improved using higher volumes of CSF, i.e. 3–5 mL. Cryptococcus grows well on most routine media, both bacterial and fungal. Primary isolation media include Sabouraud Dextrose Agar (SDA) with or without chloramphenicol, Brain Heart Infusion Agar, Staib's Birdseed Agar or Caffeic acid medium. Along with the growth of *Cryptococcus*, the latter two media turn a brownish-black due to the action of phenol oxidase resulting in the formation of melanin. Media-containing substrates for phenol oxidase facilitate recognition of *Cryptococcus* among other microorganisms in unsterile samples. *Cryptococcus* species are conventionally identified by their ability to grow at 37°C, production of enzymes urease, and phenol oxidase.

For blood cultures, both automated and lysis centrifugation methods are sensitive in detecting cryptococcemia. Blood culture positivity in HIV-infected patients has been reported to be comparatively higher (47%) than HIV-uninfected patients with CM (27%). Usually, *Cryptococcus* can be recovered in cultures within 3–7 days from untreated patients. Though not widely available, quantitative CSF cultures and its serial use has become a primary research tool for measurement of effective fungicidal activity (EFA). The quantitative yeast count has been correlated with outcomes but till date has not become a routine procedure in clinical laboratories. CSF cultures should be repeated after 2 weeks of antifungal therapy. Positive cultures signify poor outcomes and prolonged induction therapy is needed in such cases. Persistently positive CSF cultures after 4 weeks signal persistent infection.

Species identification: The two species of *Cryptococcus*, i.e. *C. neoformans* and *C. gatti,* can be differentiated by growth on a chromogenic media canavanine-glycine-bromothymol blue agar, use of kits consisting of monoclonal antibodies (presently not commercially available), commercial systems based on biochemical reactions or DNA-based analysis. Identification of *C. gatti* is important as it is associated with:

- Higher incidence of cryptococcomas
- Associated with more neurological complications, delayed response of therapy (in immunocompetent patients, may have to extend induction for 6 weeks)
- Higher incidence of neurological intervention
- Some isolates from Vancouver, Spain, Latin America have shown high azole minimum inhibitory concentrations (MICs).

Antifungal susceptibility: Antifungal susceptibility can be useful in guiding selection and monitoring of antifungal therapy, especially in cases of recurrent or persistent infection. Though methods for in vitro sensitivity testing of *Cryptococcus* have been standardized and epidemiological cut-off values have been defined.

It is recommended:

- When primary therapy fails or relapse occurs
- Previous exposure to azoles
- Cryptococcal isolates with MIC of more than or equal to 16 μg/mL for fluconazole and more than or equal to 32 μg/mL for flucytosine have been seen to be associated with relapses.

Serology

The detection of cryptococcal polysaccharide antigen in CSF, serum or plasma is an essential diagnostic tool and should be performed on CSF samples for all patients with suspected CM. Capsular polysaccharide become solubilized in the serum during infection. Serology for *Cryptococcus* diagnosis is greater than 90% sensitive and specific. Latex agglutination and ELISA (enzyme-linked immunosorbent assay) both can be used for detecting the antigen. Latex agglutination is the most common format employed for both screening and as a prognostic determinant. Latex particles coated with specific rabbit anti-*C. neoformans* antiserum are mixed with dilutions of patient CSF, serum or urine. Serum may be treated with pronase to remove inhibitory substances like rheumatoid factor. Rarely, latex agglutination assays may yield false positive results. A cross-reactive polysaccharide antigen present in *Trichosporon beigelii* may give false positive results. False positive latex agglutination tests usually have a value less than or equal to 1:8 titer. False negative results may be seen either with poorly encapsulated yeasts, low organism burden early in the course of disease and in chronic low-grade meningitis or prozone phenomenon. Most patients with AIDS have higher antigen titers than HIV uninfected patients, reflecting a higher yeast burden. Studies have established the value of latex agglutination in the diagnosis of cryptococcosis in AIDS (Figs. 13.3A and B).

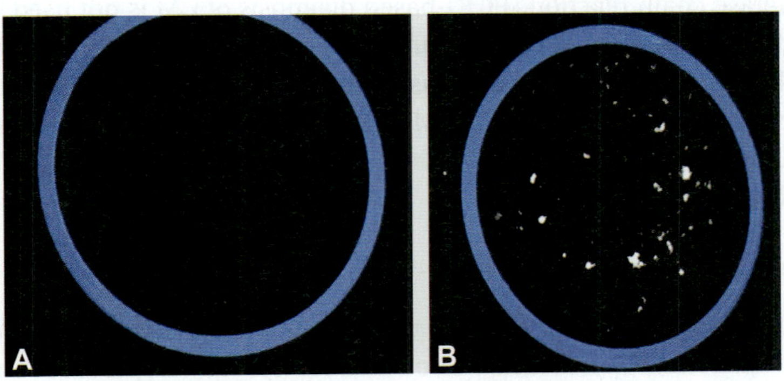

Figs. 13.3A and B: Latex agglutination test strip for *Cryptococcus*: (A) Negative and (B) Positive.

Enzyme immunoassays developed to detect cryptococcal antigen or antibodies are less subjective. They may also detect antigen earlier and in smaller amounts. Serum for enzyme immunoassay requires no pretreatment. However, these are more labor intensive and time-consuming.

A lateral flow assay (LFA) developed in 2009 is being increasingly employed as a rapid point of care test for the diagnosis of cryptococcosis. The point of care test has been validated in CSF and serum (including sampling of whole blood from finger prick) with above 99% sensitivity and specificity. It has also been tested for urine with a sensitivity of approximately 85%. LFA requires no sample pretreatment, is suitable for use in settings with minimal infrastructure, gives rapid results and is affordable. In fact, the WHO has recommended that LFA be used to screen patients with HIV infection. LFA in serum samples has recently been used as preemptive tool for diagnosing CM in HIV patients for early treatment. The use of semiquantitative LFA cryptococcal antigen titers can be used as prognostic markers as titers above 1:1,024 are associated with greater mortality at 2 and 10 weeks. Also, serum cryptococcal antigen titer more than or equal to 1:512 is a potential risk factor for cryptococcal relapse in HIV-positive patients. However, performing antigen titers can be labor intensive and very expensive. Serial cryptococcal antigen titers are also generally not helpful in predicting a treatment response as cryptococcal antigens remain elevated for a long period even when the cultures are negative. They may be of value in follow-up of HIV patients after cessation of therapy. If the titers increase and the CD4 levels decrease to less than 100 cells/μL, reinstitution of fluconazole maintenance therapy should be considered. Serial monitoring of titers should be done with the same method initially used, i.e. latex agglutination/ELISA or LFA as titers do not correlate among different methods.

Molecular Methods

Polymerase chain reaction (PCR)-based diagnosis of CM is not used widely because of availability of low cost and highly sensitive cryptococcal antigen tests. However, PCR may be used as an adjunctive method in patients with recurrent or persistent symptoms. Multiplex meningitis or encephalitis PCRs like FilmArrays System is available which can detect cryptococcal infection as early as 1 hour.

Laboratory Tests for Follow-up

Cerebrospinal fluid culture is the recommended laboratory test used for follow-up. Both India Ink examination and CSF or blood cryptococcal antigen testing are not helpful for monitoring response. The recommended timing of CSF cultures is as follows:

- *Baseline CSF culture*: Cryptococcal growth positive
- Repeat after 2 weeks for determining fungicide success of induction therapy:
  - CSF culture positive at 2 weeks: Extend the induction therapy for further 2 weeks
- Repeat CSF culture at 4 weeks. If still positive it indicates persistent infection:
  - Do antifungal susceptibility to look for any antifungal resistance.

RADIOLOGY

The radiographic appearance of CNS cryptococcosis varies according to the underlying disease and the immune status of the host. Computed tomography (CT) and magnetic resonance imaging (MRI) are the modalities of choice for the investigation of CM. MRI appears to be more sensitive than CT for detecting abnormalities. The radiographic picture markedly varies between AIDS and non-AIDS patients. Common CT scan presentations in the immunocompetent host include a normal scan (50%), hydrocephalus (25%), gyral enhancement (15%) or nodal enhancements (15%). A considerable half of HIV patients also have normal scans. However, over a third of HIV patients present with diffuse cortical atrophy. Other CT findings in AIDS include hydrocephalus and focal mass lesions. MRI findings include tiny clustered hyperintense foci on T2-weighted images and nonenhancing on postcontrast T1-weighted images within basal ganglia and midbrain representing Virchow-Robin spaces. MRI findings of dilated Virchow-Robin spaces in high-risk patients such as AIDS are highly suggestive of CM.

CONCLUSION

- Cryptococcal meningitis is the most common cause of morbidity and mortality in immunocompromised patients, especially in resource-poor settings.
- A high degree of clinical suspicion and use of appropriate diagnostic techniques are necessary for early and targeted therapy.
- India Ink preparation, cryptococcal antigen test, and CSF culture should be done in all suspected cases.
- Culture is the test of choice for follow-up of patients.
- Documentation of CSF sterilization at 2 weeks is required for discontinuation of induction therapy.
- Positive CSF cultures at 4 weeks signal persistent infection and need antifungal susceptibility testing to rule out resistance.
- A preemptive screening using LFA, a point of care tests for CM, has facilitated more rapid diagnosis of cryptococcosis especially in high-risk populations, thereby leading to better patient outcomes.

SUGGESTED READING

1. Abassi M, Boulware DR, Rhein J. Cryptococcal meningitis: diagnosis and management update. Curr Trop Med Rep. 2015;2(2):90-9.
2. Antinori S. New Insights into HIV/AIDS-associated Cryptococcosis. ISRN AIDS. 2013;2013:471363.
3. Maziarz EK, Perfect JR. Cryptococcosis. Infect Dis Clin N Am. 2016;30(2016):179-206.
4. Mitchell TG, Perfect JR. Cryptococcosis in the era of AIDS–100 years after the discovery of cryptococcus neoformans. Clin Microbiol Rev. 1995;8(4):515-48.
5. Perfect JR, Dismukes WE, Dromer F, et al. Clinical practice guidelines for the management of cryptococcal disease: 2010 update by the infectious diseases society of America. Clin Infect Dis. 2010;50(3):291-322.
6. Perfect JR. Cryptococcosis (Cryptococcus neoformans and Cryptococcus gattii). In: Bennett JE, Dolin R, Blaser MJ (Eds). Mandell, Douglas, and Bennett's Principles and Practice of Infectious Diseases, 8th edition. New York: Elsevier Saunders; 2015. pp. 2934-48.
7. Satishchandra P, Mathew T, Gadre G, et al. Cryptococcal meningitis: clinical, diagnostic and therapeutic overviews. Neurol India. 2007;55(3):226-32.

CHAPTER

14

Treatment of Cryptococcal Meningitis

Jaswinder Kaur Oberoi, Atul Kakar

INTRODUCTION

Early detection of cryptococcal meningitis is essential to improve outcome. A dipstick test for early detection of cryptococcal infection is available commercially. Cryptococcal antigen (CrAg) is serum and can be detected at least 3 weeks before symptoms of meningitis. The test should be done in all asymptomatic patients with CD4 cell counts less than 100 cells/μL. The level of CrAg can be done in both blood and CSF. Positive CrAg test is a strong indicator of disease, however CSF analysis should be done to confirm diagnosis. The lumbar puncture findings are that opening pressure usually high. The cell count is high and lymphocytic, glucose is low and protein is high. India ink and culture are useful in confirming the diagnosis as mentioned in earlier chapter.

HUMAN IMMUNODEFICIENCY-INFECTED INDIVIDUALS

The goal of treatment in cryptococcal infections is to reduce the burden of yeasts rapidly and efficiently. The guidelines of the Infectious Diseases Society of America (IDSA) for management of cryptococcal meningitis (CM) 2010, divides the treatment into three distinct phases based on several randomized control trials.

1. Induction therapy
2. Consolidation therapy
3. Maintenance therapy.

Induction therapy aims to achieve rapid cerebrospinal fluid (CSF) sterilization by using a fungicidal combination of drugs. Consolidation and maintenance therapy involve the use of fluconazole in the suppressive regimen. According to the IDSA recommendations, the treatment protocol of CM as given in Flowchart 14.1.

The CNS infection may or may not be associated with pulmonary disease.

Flowchart 14.1: Treatment protocol of cryptococcal meningitits.

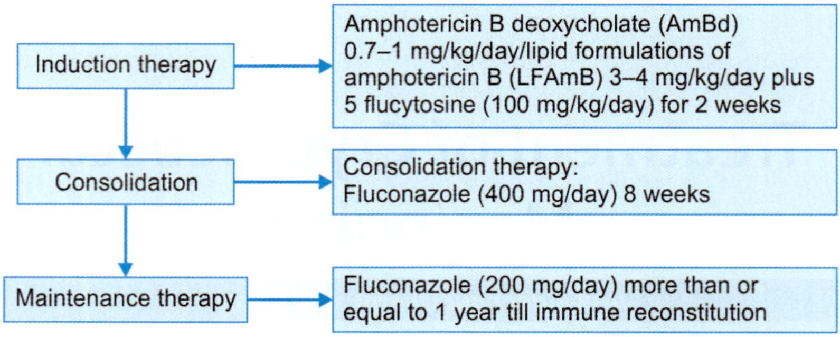

Studies have suggested elevated intracranial pressure in cryptococcal meningitis. This has been associated with increased mortality. The therapeutic lumbar puncture has been suggested to improve survival and decrease neurological complications (cranial nerve palsy, deafness, blindness etc.). Mannitol, acetazolamide, dexamethasone are routinely not recommended, ventriculoperitoneal shunt should be done if clinically indicated.

Along with aggressive antifungal therapy, management of the acute cerebral edema and increased intracranial pressure is crucial as is the decision to commence anti-retro viral therapy (ART) in human immunodeficiency (HIV) patients with CM. A delay in ART is associated with an increased mortality due to HIV and related infections. However, early commencement risks the onset of severe and fatal immune reconstitution inflammatory syndrome (IRIS) associated with an unsterilized CSF. Consensus guidelines offer options to initiate ART between 4 weeks and 6 weeks after antifungal therapy.

Persistent and relapsed infections: Positive CSF cultures after 1 month of antifungal therapy signal persistent disease. CM relapse or microbiological relapse is indicated by the recurrence of meningeal symptoms with the isolation of organisms on CSF culture after initial improvement and CSF sterilization. These should be differentiated from cryptococcal IRIS where the cultures are sterile. Management includes reinitiating induction therapy with amphotericin and higher doses of fluconazole (800–1200 mg/day). Voriconazole may be used as salvage therapy in refractory cases.

Immune Reconstitution Inflammatory Syndrome

Restoration of pathogen-specific immunity can lead to cryptococcalIRIS which is associated with clinical deterioration of the disease or a new presentation of cryptococcal disease. IRIS occurs due to the strong pro-inflammatory T helper response leading to a cytokine cascade. Cryptococcal IRIS is most commonly seen in acquired immunodeficiency syndrome (AIDS) with CM and to a lesser extent solid organ transplant recipients (incidence 5–15%) and following treatment with monoclonal antibodies such as adalimumab and alemtuzumab. Suggested criteria for IRIS include new appearance/ worsening of the clinicoradiological manifestations with an inflammatory process within 12 months of starting ART (with concomitant CD4 recovery), histopathology showing granulomas and negative results of cultures or stable or reduced biomarkers. Cryptococcal IRIS is of two varieties:

- Paradoxical IRIS in patients with a prior diagnosis of cryptococcal infection in whom ART has been started.
    - Its incidence ranges from 4.2 event/100 person-years (PY) in France to 25 events/100 PY in South Africa.
    - It can be prevented by delaying initiation of ART till 4–6 weeks of antifungal treatment.
- Anti-retro viral therapy-associated IRIS where there is unmasking of cryptococcal infection in an AIDS patient after starting ART.
    - The incidence is lower—0.2–1.6%
    - It can be prevented by preemptive screening for serum cryptococcal capsular antigen in HIV patients with CD4 less than100 cells/μL before starting ART.

PROGNOSIS AND OUTCOME

Cryptococcal meningitis if untreated is a fatal disease. Even with antifungal treatment, the outcomes depend upon the host presentation, underlying diseases and the nature of the pathogen. Poorer outcomes have been seen to be associated with CM under the following conditions:

- Abnormal mental status
- High CSF fungal burden (high cryptococcal antigen titers ≥ 1:1024)
- Disseminated disease (particularly seen in AIDS patients)
- Wasting syndrome (low body mass index)
- Symptoms of elevated intracranial pressure
- Low CSF leukocyte counts
- Lack of flucytosine treatment during induction phase
- Induction treatment with low dose fluconazole.

PREVENTION

As CM carries a high mortality especially in resource constrained settings, a "screen and treat" approach is advocated by the WHO wherein serum cryptococcal antigen testing followed by preemptive fluconazole therapy in ART-naïve adults with a CD4 count of less than 100 cells/μL is recommended in endemic settings.

CONCLUSION

Most patients with CM have CD4 cells less than 100 cells/μL

- Anphotericin-B, azoles and 5-flucytorine are drugs effective against cryptococcal.
- Mortality rates of cryptococcal infection in HIV patient is 20%.
- Raise intracranial pressure is associated with raised mortality. Dexamethasone therapy is associated with more mortality whereas repeated lumbar punctures is associated with less mortality.
- ART should be delayed till indication therapy is completed.
- No vaccine is available for cryptococcal infection primary prophylaxis with fluconazole (200 mg/dL) is effective in reducing prevalence of this disease.

SUGGESTED READING

1. Lofgen S, Mahsa A, Joshua R, et al. Recent advances in AIDS-related cryptococcal meningitis treatment with an emphasis on resource limited settings. Expert Rev Anti Infect Ther. 2017;15:331-40.
2. Makadzange AT, McHugh G. New approaches to the diagnosis and treatment of cryptococcal meningitis. Semin Neurol. 2014;34:47-60.
3. Njei B, Kongnyuy EJ, Kumar S, et al. Optimal timing for antiretroviral therapy initiation in patients with HIV infection and concurrent cryptococcal meningitis. Cochrane Database Syst Rev. 2013;2:CD009012.
4. Yao ZW, Lu X, Shen C, et al. Comparison of flucytosine and flueonazole combined with amphotericin B for the treatment of HIV-associated cryptococcal meningitis: a systematic review and meta-analysis. Eur J Clin Microbiol Infect Dir. 2014;33(8): 1339-44.

CHAPTER 15

Pneumocystis jirovecii in Human Immunodeficiency Virus

Bobby Bhalotra

INTRODUCTION

Pneumocystis carinii pneumonitis (PCP) is a common opportunistic disease that occurs almost exclusively in patients who have a profound immunodeficiency state. It is one of the leading causes of life-threatening opportunistic infection in human immunodeficiency virus (HIV) patients who have low CD4 cell counts. The name *Pneumocystis carinii* has undergone slight alteration and is now referred to as *Pneumocystis jirovecii* (PCJ).

Apart from HIV patients the other subsets of population at substantial risk of developing this infection are those with malignancies (particularly hematological cancers) and patients on glucocorticoids, chemotherapeutic and immunosuppressive medications. The hematopoietic stem cell and solid organ transplant recipients are also at a high risk of this infection.

MICROBIOLOGY

As *P. jirovecii* organisms are atypical fungi, they do not grow in fungal culture. They have a cell wall that contains cholesterol rather than ergosterol. The life cycle consists of the trophic form, a precystic form, and the cystic form. The trophic form predominates over the cystic form during infection. They atypically respond to some antiparasitic agents.

PATHOGENESIS

Transmission

The primary mode of transmission of *P. jirovecii* is via the airborne route. The infection occurs early in life, with 75% of humans infected by the age of 4 years.

Pathogen-host interaction determines the possibility of clinical disease. Pneumocystis exists almost exclusively within the alveoli of the lung. Immune control of Pneumocystis involves production of chemokines and inflammatory cytokines by alveolar macrophages and epithelial cells. The macrophages in the alveoli of the lungs are the primary phagocytes which will mediate the clearance of these organisms from the body. Phagocytosis and the inflammatory activation of alveolar macrophages in response to Pneumocystis are impaired in HIV-infected persons and contribute to the genesis of infection in this subset of population.

Healthy individuals, as well as those with HIV infection, may harbor Pneumocystis in their respiratory tract and may be completely asymptomatic. The prevalence of Pneumocystis colonization among healthy adults ranges from 0 to 20%.

Incidence

There has been a dramatic decline in the incidence of PCP after the advent of the potent anti-retro viral therapy (ART).

Risk Factors

The main risk factor for PCP is advanced immunosuppression in patients not taking ART.

Other risk factors include:

- CD4 count less than 200 cells/μL
- CD4 cell percentage less than 14%
- Previous history of any episode of PCP or recurrent bacterial pneumonia in a patient
- High HIV RNA plasma levels
- Oral thrush
- History of substantial weight loss.

CLINICAL FEATURES OF PULMONARY DISEASE

Approximately 5–10% of patients are asymptomatic.

The onset of the disease is gradual and subacute. Patients often complain of the classical triad of a dry cough subfebrile temperature and dyspnea on exertion. The illness worsens over days to weeks but a fulminant pneumonia is an uncommon finding. Fatigue, chills, and weight loss are also important symptoms to watch for.

Physical examination usually reveals fever, tachypnea, tachycardia, and hypoxemia. Many patients have thrush and weight loss. Auscultation of the chest may be normal or diffuse dry rales are heard. Pulse oximetry reveals oxygen desaturation on walking or exercising and it is highly suggestive of a diagnosis of PCP. Oral thrush is a very common coinfection.

Extrapulmonary disease is seen rarely. It can occur in any organ and is usually associated with aerosolized-pentamidine prophylaxis.

DIAGNOSIS

Clinical presentation of atypical pneumonia in the setting of HIV may be suggestive but definitive diagnosis should be sought for. The main problem arises is the organism cannot be cultured. An array of investigations can be performed to help reach a diagnosis. They are:

Laboratory Findings

- *Low CD4 counts*: The CD4 count usually drops below 200 cells/µL with a cell percentage less than 14.
- *Oxygenation*: Hypoxia occurs with progression of PCP. The alveolar-arterial oxygen gradient is widened in more than 90% of patients and ranges from mild (alveolar-arterial O_2 difference < 35 mm Hg) to severe (alveolar-arterial O_2 difference > 45 mm Hg).
- *Lactate dehydrogenase levels*: Despite appropriate treatment, if the lactate dehydrogenase (LDH) level continues to increase, it is a poor prognostic marker.
- *Diffusion lung capacity for carbon monoxide*: If the diffusion lung capacity for carbon monoxide (DLCO) is within normal limits (i.e. within 70% of the predicted value or greater), it is highly unlikely that the patient has PCP.
- *C-reactive protein*: It is normal provided the patient does not have any other infection.

Radiography

Chest Radiographs

Approximately 25% of the patients with PCP have a normal chest radiograph. The rest may show diffuse, bilateral, interstitial, or alveolar infiltrates. Upper lobe involvement is commonly seen. Pneumatoceles and a pneumothorax can also be present in some cases.

High-resolution Computed Tomography

The presence of patchy or nodular ground-glass attenuation in high-resolution computed tomography (HRCT) is used to diagnose possible PCP in suspected patients. HRCT has a specificity of 89% and a sensitivity of 100% whereas a normal resolution CT may fail to pick up the disease. The findings are perihilar (butterfly shaped) interstitial infiltrates.

Microbiology

The diagnosis relies upon the visualization of the cystic or trophic forms in appropriate specimens, since Pneumocystis cannot be cultured.

Stains that have commonly been used include Gomori-methenamine silver. Immunofluorescent staining using fluorescein-labeled monoclonal antibodies is the preferred technique as it picks up a greater percentage of cases.

Specimens for microbiology can be obtained by various techniques:

- *Induced sputum and bronchoalveolar lavage*: Sputum induction is done by the use of nebulized hypertonic saline. Although it is a useful method to obtain an adequate sample, bronchoalveolar lavage (BAL) is a more sensitive technique.

  It has a better diagnostic yield amounting to 90–100% in HIV-infected patients.
- *Tissue biopsy is needed only when* sputum induction and BAL are nondiagnostic.

  Tissues are obtained by performing transbronchial lung biopsies during bronchoscopies or by video-assisted lung biopsies.
- *Endotracheal aspirates*: In patients who are intubated and mechanically ventilated, endotracheal aspirates can be taken for detection of PCP. They have a high sensitivity so this is the preferred method in these patients.

PRESUMPTIVE DIAGNOSIS

There are times when a definitive diagnosis cannot be made due to a low burden of organisms and/or the inability to obtain the necessary specimen. In those situations, a decision must be made whether or not to continue treatment.

Clinical and radiographic findings can be highly suggestive of a diagnosis of PCP in HIV-infected patients who are having a low CD4 cell count. Increasingly, elevated levels of 1-3-beta-d-glucan are also used to help support this diagnosis.

DIFFERENTIAL DIAGNOSIS

The differential diagnosis of PCP includes:

- Pneumonia due to bacteria, fungi, viruses, and mycobacteria. Most common infections are tuberculosis, nontuberculous mycobacteria, histoplasmosis, toxoplasmosis, cytomegalovirus (CMV), and primary influenza pneumonia.
- Acute bronchitis
- Neoplasm
- Drug hypersensitivity
- Pulmonary hypertension
- Cardiomyopathy
- Kaposi's sarcoma.

Prophylaxis—Primary Prophylaxis

The indications for primary prophylaxis are:

- Any HIV patient with CD4 counts less than 200 cells/mm^3 or who have a history of oropharyngeal candidiasis or CD4 cell percentage of less than 14% should receive chemoprophylaxis against PCP. This includes all HIV infected patients on ART and pregnant women as well.
- Any person with a history of an acquired immunodeficiency syndrome (AIDS)-defining illness.
- Any patient with a CD4 counts between 200 cells/mm^3 and 250 cells/mm^3 who is unable to come for regular follow-up, i.e. get his CD4 count monitored every 3 months.

The recommended prophylactic agents to be used are trimethoprim and sulfamethoxazole combination (TMP-SMX). They are to be taken in a daily dose of one double-strength tablet. Alternative prophylactic regimens are available for patients who are unable to tolerate a TMP-SMX regime. They include: dapsone, pyrimethamine, leucovorin, and aerosolized pentamidine.

In those patients who have an increase in CD4 counts to values greater than 200 cells/mm^3 within 3 months of treatment and who have shown a response to ART, the primary prophylaxis should be discontinued. If the CD4 count falls back to values less than 200 cells/mm^3 any time during the course of illness, the prophylaxis can again be reintroduced.

Treatment

The treatment of choice for all *Pneumocystis carinii* pneumonia cases is the combination of TMP-SMX. The therapy is guided according to the severity of the disease and the doses of the medication should be adjusted according to the renal function of the patient.

For all HIV patients with PCP, having a mild-to-moderate disease, a combination of TMP-SMX given on an outpatient basis is highly effective. New patients with moderate-to-severe illness should be administered corticosteroids along with the specific PCP therapy. This adjuvant steroid therapy should be started at the earliest or within 72 hours. These patients need ICU care and have an overall poor prognosis.

There are alternative regimens also available. They include therapy with dapsone and TMP, primaquine plus clindamycin and atovaquone in people with mild-to-moderate illness. For patients with moderate-to-severe disease therapies available apart from the conventional ones are treatment with combinations of clindamycin and primaquine or with pentamidine given intravenously. Before starting on dapsone or primaquine, it is essential that the patient should undergo a test to rule out glucose-6-phosphate dehydrogenase (G6PD) deficiency. The therapy should be continued for a period of 21 days as per recommendations.

Most HIV patients are on ART. If not ART should initiated in all the patients of HIV with PCP at the earliest or within 2 weeks of diagnosis. It is essential to monitor for an adequate response to therapy and look for adverse effects due to the various drugs being used as these patients are highly immunosuppressed.

Adverse Events after Therapy

The rate of adverse effects after therapy in AIDS patients is significantly high. The most commonly seen reactions with TMP-SMX are fever, cytopenias like leukopenia and thrombocytopenia, rashes, including Stevens-Johnson syndrome, renal and hepatic dysfunction, and hyperkalemia. The alternative therapy also has an array of adverse reactions which includes:

- Primaquine/dapsone—methemoglobinemia and hemolysis (especially in patients with G6PD deficiency)
- Dapsone—fever and rashes
- Pentamidine—pancreatitis with episodes of hypo- and hyperglycemias, leukopenia, azotemia with electrolyte abnormalities and cardiac dysrhythmias
- Primaquine and clindamycin—fever, anemia, rashes, and diarrhea
- Atovaquone—elevation of transaminases, headache, nausea, and diarrhea
- Paradoxical immune reconstitution inflammatory syndrome (IRIS) has been reported following PCP. Most cases have occurred within weeks of the episode of PCP.

Failure of Treatment

If there is lack of improvement or there is further deterioration of the pulmonary function of the patient according to the arterial blood gas analysis even after he has received anti-PCP therapy for a period of at least 4–8 days, it is defined as clinical or treatment failure. It occurs in around 10% of cases with mild-to-moderate disease and is usually attributed to lack of drug efficacy. It is essential to exclude all other coexisting infections before labeling a case as that of clinical failure and a bronchoscopy with BAL can be performed to help in reaching a conclusion.

In around one-third of patients, the toxicity and adverse reactions due to drugs may attribute to the treatment failure.

Secondary Prophylaxis

Chemoprophylaxis should be given for life in all patients of HIV who have a history of PCP with TMP-SMX. This is referred to as secondary prophylaxis. It should be discontinued if the CD4 counts increase to numbers greater than 200 cells/mm^3 in less than 3 months of initiating the ART. Prophylaxis can be reintroduced in such cases if the CD4 count again falls below the critical limit of 200 cells/mm^3 at any point of time.

If the patient develops PCP with a CD4 count greater than 200 cells/mm^3, it becomes prudent here to continue PCP prophylaxis for life. The rise in CD4 cell count as a consequence of ART is nonconsequential in such cases.

CONCLUSION

- *Pneumocystis jirovecii* pneumonia is life-threatening if not recognized and treated.
- *Pneumocystis jirovecii* pneumonia primarily involves the lungs; extrapulmonary presentations are very rare.
- Suspected cases should receive treatment immediately even in the presence of a normal radiograph.
- High-resolution computed tomography may demonstrate perihilar infiltrates in classical cases.
- Hypoxemia on arterial blood gas analysis (ABGA), elevated LSH are other tests which may suggest PCJ.
- Co-trimoxazole is the drug of choice given for 21 days in a dose of 960 mg tablets thrice daily. In severe disease, intravenous medication should be considered.
- Prednisolone is indicated as clinical deterioration may occur when the Pneumocystis bursts. The dose of prednisolone is 1 mg/kg for 5–10 days. All patients with altered ABGA should also receive this.
- The incidence of PCP is very low on patients receiving prophylaxis.
- *Pneumocystis carinii* pneumonitis may present just with fever, weight loss, and fatigue.

SUGGESTED READING

1. Akgün KM, Pisani M, Crothers K. The changing epidemiology of HIV-infected patients in the intensive care unit. J Intens Care Med. 2011;26(3):151-64.
2. Siegel M, Masur H, Kovacs J. Pneumocystis jirovecii pneumonia in human immunodeficiency virus infection. Semin Respir Crit Care Med. 2016;37(2):243-56.
3. Sokulska M, Kicia M, Wesołowska M. Pneumocystis jirovecii—from a commensal to pathogen: clinical and diagnostic review. Parasitol Res. 2015;114(10):3577-85.
4. Tasaka S, Tokuda H. Recent advances in the diagnosis of Pneumocystis jirovecii pneumonia in HIV-infected adults. Expert Opin Med Diagn. 2013;7(1):85-97.
5. Wang RJ, Miller RF, Huang L. Approach to fungal infections in human immunodeficiency virus-infected individuals. Clin Chest Med. 2017;38(3):465-77.

SECTION 6

Special Problems

CHAPTER 16

HIV-associated Nephropathy

Vinant Bhargava, Lovy Gaur

HIV-ASSOCIATED KIDNEY DISEASE

The human immunodeficiency virus (HIV) is associated with both acute kidney injury (AKI) and chronic kidney disease (CKD). HIV-associated kidney disease, classically known as HIV-associated nephropathy (HIVAN), was first described in 1984 and occurs due to the acquired immunodeficiency syndrome (AIDS) (Flowchart 16.1). HIVAN may occur in patients with acute seroconversion and also in patients with less advanced HIV infection. Evaluating a patient with HIVAN is similar to any patient evaluated for renal failure. This includes a detailed history focusing on medications and infections, physical examination, urine examination of sediment, blood and urine chemistries and kidney imaging studies. Kidney biopsy is indicated in those with AKI without a clear cause, especially with a nephritic sediment; nephritis or proteinuria and clinical evidence of thrombotic microangiopathy.

Flowchart 16.1: HIV and kidney

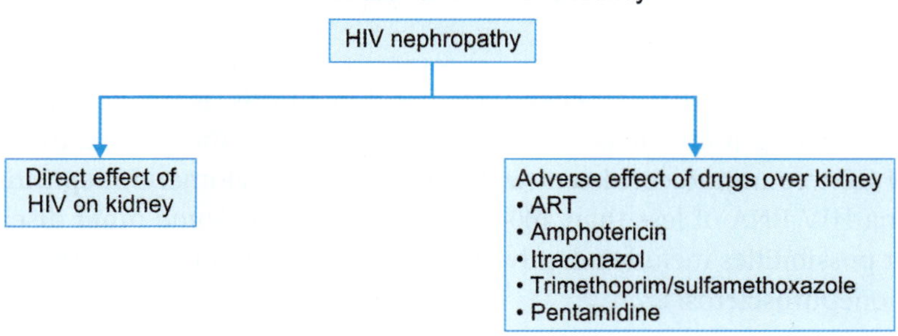

GLOMERULAR DISORDERS

HIV-associated Collapsing Glomerulopathy

Pathogenesis

Viral factors: Specific HIV accessory proteins such as Vpr and Nef have been shown to damage renal cells independent of directly infecting them.

Experimental transgenic mice models have suggested that the expression of these proteins in podocytes is associated with progressive disease, loss of podocyte differentiation markers as well as features suggestive of collapsing glomerulopathy and segmental glomerulosclerosis. Collapsing glomerulopathy is characterized by nephrotic proteinuria.

Host factors: Individuals of African descent are 20 times more predilection to developed glomerulonephritis; this may be linked to genetic polymorphism in the *MYH9* gene encoding myosin heavy chain 9. Another important gene implicated is APOL1 encoding apolipoprotein L1. APOL1 codon changing variants confer an odds ratio of 29. Homozygosity for two risk alleles (G1 and G2) has been observed in approximately 50% of African Americans with HIV-associated CG, compared with only 12% of African American controls. It is interesting to note that these variants appear to protect individuals from African sleeping sickness caused by *Trypanosoma brucei* rhodesiense.

Clinical Manifestations

Patients present with proteinuria and renal impairment. Edema is less frequent than with other conditions causing nephrotic range proteinuria. Some patients present with uremia. Radiological imaging may reveal an increased kidney size despite reduced glomerular filtration rate.

Pathology

HIV-associated glomerulonephritis is indistinguishable from other causes of glomerulonephritis. Features include proliferation of podocytes, collapse of the glomerular tuft, microtubular cystic changes and intracytoplasmic tubuloreticular inclusions with dilated cisterns of the endoplasmic reticulum.

Diagnosis

The diagnosis of HIV-associated glomerulonephritis is made by renal biopsy. Among individuals of African descent, nephritic proteinuria and a low CD4 count are consistent with HIV-associated glomerulonephritis; a plasma HIV RNA of less than 400 copies/mL suggests some other disease. Other possibilities include adaptive focal segmental glomerulosclerosis and arterionephrosclerosis.

Treatment

The HIVAN is an indication for initiation of ART regardless of the T-lymphocyte count. The DART study (development of anti retroviral therapy) conducted in Uganda and Zimbabwe demonstrated an improvement in kidney function of 2–6 mL/min/1.73 m^2 after 4–5 years of ART. Treatment with combination anti-retro viral therapy has lowered the incidence of end-stage renal disease (ESRD) in HIVAN.

Treatment also includes control of blood pressure to a level below 130/80 mm Hg and preferable use of angiotensin-converting enzyme inhibitors and angiotensin II receptor blockers.

Natural History

In HIV infected patients, progression of CKD is more rapid in those of African American descent probably reflecting the effect of APOL1 variants. Predictors of progression are a high degree of chronic damage on histology, severe renal dysfunction at baseline, high grade proteinuria and the presence of a large number of sclerotic glomeruli. Concomitant use of renin-angiotensin blockade results in improved survival.

HIV-associated Immune Complex Glomerulonephritis

Immune complex glomerulonephritis is commoner in those of European and Asian ancestry, suffering from HIV. In some cases, immune complexes include HIV antigens; other cases may represent polyclonal B-cell expansion that accompanies HIV disease. Clinically, the subjects may present with nephritic range proteinuria and hematuria. Biopsy may reveal mesangial proliferative glomerulonephritis or focal or diffuse glomerulonephritis with endocapillary proliferation. Immune deposits may be seen in the mesangium andsubendothelial or subepithelial regions. Patients with hepatitis C coinfection may manifest with membranoproliferative glomerulonephritis.

Arterionephrosclerosis

Chronic HIV infection is associated with premature ageing. This may manifest as arterionephrosclerosis, which is characterized by—arterial intimal thickening, medial hypertrophy and duplication of the internal elastic lamina together with global glomerulosclerosis. These findings are also typically seen in patients with hypertension.

Tubular Disorders

There are several tubular disorders associated with HIV infection. The majority of these are secondary to drugs commonly used in the treatment of HIV. Proximal tubular injury manifests as glycosuria, phosphaturia, uricosuria, proteinuria and aminoaciduria. Diabetes insipidus is suggestive of distal tubular involvement. The most common drug causing tubular injury is tenofovir. Risk factors for tenofovir induced nephrotoxicity include a low CD4 count, previous history of renal impairment, and combination therapy with didanosine and protease inhibitors (lopinavir and ritonavir). Other protease inhibitors, nucleotide and nucleoside reverse transcriptase inhibitors have variable effects on tubular function. Indinavir is associated with crystalluria.

RENAL REPLACEMENT THERAPY IN PATIENT WITH HIV INFECTION

Hemodialysis

The HIV/AIDS patients do not have to be isolated from other patients or dialyzed on separate machines. However, the concerns of staff and patients results in these patients being dialyzed in separate facilities in a few dialysis centers. Reprocessing of dialyzers from HIV-positive patients does not place staff members at a risk of infection provided that necessary sterile precautions are followed.

Peritoneal Dialysis

The HIV virus can survive in peritoneal effluents for up to 7 days and in peritoneal dialysis exchange tubing for 48 hour sand these intervals are effective in killing HIV in the dialysate. Sodium hypochlorite (50% solution) and household bleach (10% solution), each further diluted to 1:512 are used.

Kidney Transplantation

Kidney transplantation is the most definite means for renal replacement therapy. Patients undergoing kidney transplantation have survival rates similar to those of HIV uninfected patients. There is no increased risk of opportunistic infections noted in the HIV kidney transplant patients. In spite of high rates of acute cellular rejection, survival is similar to noninfected persons.

Dose Adjustment of Anti-retro Viral Drugs

Nucleoside/nucleotide analogs

Drug	*Standard dosage*	*Dosing in chronic kidney disease and hemodialysis*	
Zidovudine	300 mg PO BID	Creatinine clearance (mL/min)	
		<15	100 mg Q 6-8 H
		HD	100 mg TID
Tenofovir	300 mg PO QD	Creatinine clearance (mL/min)	
		≥50	300 mg QD
		30–49	300 mg Q 48 H
		10–29	300 mg twice weekly (i.e. Q 3–4 days)
		HD	300 mg QW
Lamivudine	150 mg PO BID or 300 mg PO QD	Creatinine clearance (mL/min)	
		≥50	150 mg BID or 300 mg QD
		30–49	150 mg QD
		15–29	150 mg first dose, then 100 mg QD
		5–14	150 mg first dose, then 50 mg QD
		<5	50 mg first dose, then 25 mg QD

Emtricitabine	200 mg PO QD	Creatinine clearance (mL/min)	
		≥50	200 mg QD
		30–49	200 mg Q 48 H
		15–29	200 mg Q 72 H
		<15	200 mg Q 96 H
		HD	200 mg Q 96 H, give dose after dialysis

Nonnucleoside reverse transcriptase inhibitors

Drug(s)	***Management***	***References***
Nevirapine	*For patients with chronic kidney disease (not on hemodialysis)*: Dosage adjustment does not appear necessary *For patients on hemodialysis*: An additional 200 mg dose of nevirapine following each dialysis treatment is recommended.	Viramune package insert

Protease inhibitors

Drug(s)	***Management***	***References***
Amprenavir, atazanavir, darunavir, fosamprenavir, indinavir, lopinavir/ritonavir, nelfinavir, ritonavir, saquinavir, tipranavir	*For patients with chronic kidney disease (not on hemodialysis)*: Dosage adjustment does not appear necessary.	
Atazanavir	Although atazanavir is not cleared by hemodialysis, patients on hemodialysis have substantially lower plasma atazanavir concentrations compared with controls. Unboosted atazanavir should not be used. For treatment-naïve patients receiving hemodialysis, atazanavir must be boosted by ritonavir. For treatment-experienced patients receiving hemodialysis, atazanavir (boosted or unboosted) is not recommended.	Reyataz package insert
Lopinavir/ritonavir	Lopinavir and ritonavir also are not cleared by hemodialysis, but a recent study found that levels of both agents were lower than those of historical controls (C_{min} was 44% lower). Dosage adjustments have not been studied. Exercise caution in patients with resistance to protease inhibitors; lopinavir and ritonavir levels may not be adequate for viral suppression.	

Chemokine coreceptor antagonists

Drug(s)	*Management*	*References*
Maraviroc	Dosage adjustment for patients with mild or moderate chronic kidney disease does not appear necessary. Maraviroc should not be used in patients with severe renal impairment or end-stage renal disease (Creatinine clearance <30 mL/min) who are taking a potent CYP3A inhibitor or inducer.	Selzentry package insert

Integrase inhibitors

Drug(s)	*Management*	*References*
Elvitegravir/ cobicistat	Do not initiate combination of elvitegravir/cobicistat/tenofovir/ emtricitabine if Creatinine clearance <70 mL/min. Discontinue if creatinine clearance decreases to <50 mL/min.	Stribild package insert

CONCLUSION

- HIV-associated nephropathy (HIVAN) was earlier called AIDS associated nephropathy. It has characteristic features of nephritic range proteinuria, kidneys are normal to large in size (on ultrasound), azotemia, normal pressure and renal biopsy has features focal segmental glomerulosclerosis (FSGS).
- HIV mediations can have effect on kidney. Tenovofir is nephrotoxic drug and protease inhibitors may precipitate nephrolithiasis, Stavudine causes hyperuricemia whereas Didanosine causes electrolyte imbalance, both these drugs are not used routinely.
- Corticosteroids on short-term use can benefit HIVAN.
- Patients who have ESRS should be offered dialysis or kidney transplant.
- Drugs like Abacavir, Delavirdine, Efavirenz, Raltegravir, Enfuvirtide and Rilpivirine does not require dose adjustment in renal failure.

SUGGESTED READING

1. Calza L, Vanino E, Magistrelli E, et al. Prevalence of renal disease within an urban HIV-infected cohort in northern Italy. Clin Exp Nephrol. 2014;18(1):104-12.
2. Dominguez S, Ghosn J, Peytavin G, et al. Efficacy and safety of tenofovir double-dose in treatment-experienced HIV-infected patients: the TENOPLUS study. J Med Virol. 2007;79(2):105-10.

3. Eustace JA, Nuermberger E, Choi M, et al. Cohort study of the treatment of severe HIV-associated nephropathy with corticosteroids. Kidney Int. 2000;58(3):1253-60.
4. Fabian J, Naicker S, Goetsch S, et al. The clinical and histological response of HIV-associated kidney disease to antiretroviral therapy in South Africans. Nephrol Dial Transplant. 2013;28(6):1543-54.
5. Foy MC, Estrella MM, Lucas GM, et al. Comparison of risk factors and outcomes in HIV immune complex kidney disease and HIV-associated nephropathy. Clin J Am Soc Nephrol. 2013;8(9):1524-32.
6. Ifudu O, Rao TK, Tan CC, et al. Zidovudine is beneficial in human immunodeficiency virus associated nephropathy. Am J Nephrol. 1995; 15(3):217-21.
7. Kaku M, Simpson DM. HIV neuropathy. Curr Opin HIV AIDS. 2014;9(6):521-6.
8. Locke JE, Montgomery RA, Warren DS, et al. Renal transplant in HIV-positive patients: long-term outcomes and risk factors for graft loss. Arch Surg. 2009;144(1):83-6.
9. Pillay P, Wadley AL, Cherry CL, et al. Pharmacological treatment of painful HIV-associated sensory neuropathy. S Afr Med J. 2015;105 (9):769-72.
10. Rockwood N, Mandalia S, Bower M, et al. Ritonavir-boosted atazanavir exposure is associated with an increased rate of renal stones compared with efavirenz, ritonavir-boosted lop-inavir and ritonavir-boosted darunavir. AIDS. 2011;25(13):1671-3.
11. Smith MC, Austen JL, Carey JT, et al. Prednisone improves renal function and proteinuria in human immunodeficiency virus-associated nephropathy. Am J Med. 1996;101(1):41-8.
12. Wei A, Burns GC, Williams BA. Long-term renal survival in HIV-associated nephropathy with angio-tensin-converting enzyme inhibition. Kidney Int. 2003;64(4):1462-71.
13. Wyatt CM, Morgello S, Katz-Malamed R, et al. The spectrum of kidney disease in patients with AIDS in the era of antiretroviral therapy. Kidney Int. 2009;75(4):428-34.

CHAPTER

17

Endocrinal Manifestations of HIV Infection

Kunal Chawla

"What the mind does not know, the eyes do not see."

INTRODUCTION

With improving management protocols and increased survival of patients with human immunodeficiency virus (HIV) infection, physicians treating such patients pay great attention and care toward management of the primary disease. Excellent guidelines are in place for screening and management of the various opportunistic infections but what is sorely lacking is an endocrinological surveillance protocol. Patients with HIV have a high incidence of problems like adrenal insufficiency, hypogonadism, thyroid dysfunction, insulin resistance and diabetes. While these endocrinopathies may be due to the primary disease, the theories for their etiopathogenesis have been steadily expanding to include treatment-related endocrine dysfunction. These medication-related endocrinopathies are increasingly being seen due to better overall disease control and survival with improved treatment regimens. In this chapter, we will be discussing the various endocrinopathies encountered in patients with HIV/acquired immunodeficiency syndrome (AIDS) (Fig. 17.1).

ADRENAL GLAND

Adrenal Insufficiency

The adrenal gland is the most common endocrine organ to be found abnormal on autopsy in a patient who has died of AIDS. The pathologies of the adrenals that have been reported on postmortem examination include infections by cytomegalovirus (CMV), *Myobacteria tuberculosis* (including atypical mycobacteria), cryptococcus, Toxoplasma, Pneumocystis as well as noninfectious causes like Kaposi sarcoma, lymphoma and adrenal hemorrhage.

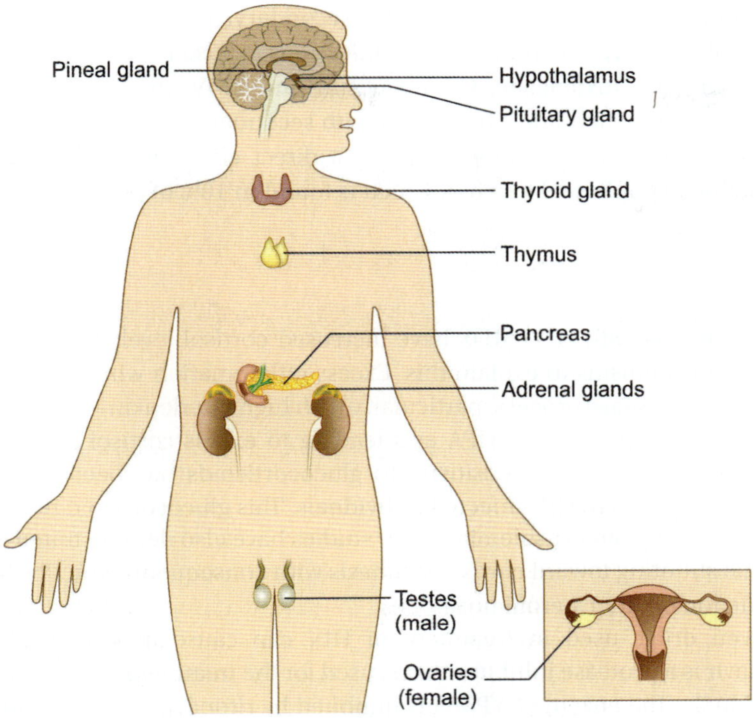

Fig. 17.1: Endocrine manifestations of HIV infection.

In spite of so many pathologies affecting the adrenal gland, overt adrenal insufficiency is rare and clinical features of the same have been reported in studies to the extent of only 4%. This is due to the fact that at least 90% of the adrenals need to be affected to produce clinical adrenal insufficiency. The most common pathogen to affect the adrenals, CMV usually destroys about 50–60% of the adrenal glands.

Even though overt and clinically manifesting adrenal insufficiency is rare, subclinical insufficiency is much more common in patients with HIV/AIDS and studies have demonstrated that about 17% of all patients with HIV/AIDS are thus affected. This insufficiency can be detected by a suboptimal cortisol response (<18 μg/dL) to stimulation with synthetic adrenocorticotropic hormone (ACTH; the Synacthen test).

Various drugs used for treatment of HIV or the opportunistic infections associated with it are also known to cause adrenal insufficiency. Ketoconazole and Itraconazole impair adrenal steroidogenesis, Rifampin increases cortisol metabolism while Megestrol acetate, a synthetic progestational derivative used as an appetite stimulant and for HIV wasting, has glucocorticoid properties and decreases ACTH. This drug suppresses the hypothalamic-pituitary-adrenal (HPA) axis and causes adrenal insufficiency if withdrawn abruptly.

Adrenal insufficiency can also be secondary, i.e. due to pituitary or hypothalamic dysfunction. Some infections caused by opportunistic pathogens like Toxoplasma Cryptococcus, and CMV are known to cause pituitary dysfunction and can present with secondary adrenal insufficiency. Another entity which is thought to be a direct effect of the HIV virus is idiopathic hypophyseal necrosis which is found in 10% of people with AIDS on autopsy.

Hypercortisolemia

Some patients with HIV/AIDS have increased cortisol levels and there are several mechanisms to explain this. Excess inflammation which is a part of the primary disease process, particularly with high interleukin-6 (IL-6) levels is known to stimulate the HPA axis leading to excess cortisol production. Additionally, decreased sensitivity to glucocorticoids has been shown in the immune cells of HIV-infected individuals. This glucocorticoid resistance also leads to hypercortisolemia. Other studies have also demonstrated intra-adrenal shunting toward cortisol synthesis with consequent reduction in the production of other steroid hormones.

Even drugs used in treatment of HIV can cause hypercortisolemia. Ritonavir is a protease inhibitor that is used for the treatment of HIV-infected individuals. The enzyme CYP3A4 is inhibited by ritonavir and consequently the metabolism of many drugs is affected. Corticosteroids used in patients on Ritonavir, even in low doses or inhaled/topical forms, can cause iatrogenic Cushing's syndrome due to the accumulation of steroids secondary to a reduced CYP3A4-mediated metabolism. Abrupt withdrawal of corticosteroids in such patients can lead to HPA axis suppression and adrenal insufficiency.

Who should be Checked for Adrenal Function and How should they be Evaluated?

The test of choice for evaluating adrenal function is the Synacthen test. This is a test in which 250 µg of intravenous corticotropin is administered and the serum cortisol levels are checked 30 and 60 minutes later. A peak cortisol level less than 18 µg/dL is suggestive of adrenal insufficiency. Once confirmed, the type of adrenal insufficiency (primary vs secondary) should be determined by checking the ACTH levels. If it is technically not possible to do the Synacthen test, we can also check a morning serum cortisol level along with an ACTH level. A morning cortisol less than 5 µg/dL suggests adrenal insufficiency.

As a guide, the following subset of patients with HIV should be considered for evaluation of their adrenal functions:

- Those with clinical features suggestive of adrenal insufficiency (postural hypotension, hyponatremia, pigmentation, etc.)
- Those with opportunistic infections or drug use known to cause adrenal insufficiency

- Disseminated CMV
- Disseminated tuberculosis
- Recent use of megestrol acetate.

If a patient with HIV/AIDS having signs and symptoms of adrenal insufficiency is found to have high levels of cortisol, we should consider the possibility of glucocorticoid resistance.

If the cortisol levels and ACTH levels are low while the patient has clinical features of cortisol excess, then exogenous steroid use should be considered. As mentioned above, even very low doses of corticosteroids can lead to iatrogenic Cushing's syndrome due to interaction with anti-retro viral drugs like ritonavir.

THYROID GLAND

"Sick Euthyroid" with a Difference

The HIV/AIDS is a severe chronic illness with a lot of adverse effects on the body. Consequently it was expected that such patients can have the usual 'sick euthyroid syndrome' with low free T3 (FT3), variable free T4 (FT4), relatively low thyroid-stimulating hormone (TSH) and high reverse T3 (rT3) levels. While abnormal thyroid function is quite common among patients with HIV/AIDS, to the extent of 16% in some studies, its pattern is different from that seen in the usual nonthyroidal illnesses. Patients with HIV/AIDS were found to have non elevated rT3 and normal T3 levels which are not seen in the usual nonthyroidal illnesses.

Autoimmune Thyroid Disease

Autoimmune thyroid disease has been found with an increasing prevalence in studies done among patients with HIV/AIDS. Both autoimmune hypothyroidism and Graves' disease are found more commonly than in the general population.

In a study by Madge et al. done in 1,565 patients with HIV/AIDS, 39 (2.5%) were found to have overt hypothyroidism, less than 1% had overt hyperthyroidism and 61 (4%) had subclinical hypothyroidism. The prevalence rate was not found to be sufficient to warrant screening of thyroid functions in every patient with HIV/AIDS.

Thyroiditis

Although rare, cases of thyroiditis have been reported with *Pneumocystis jirovecii*, *Cryptococcus neoformans*, visceral leishmaniasis, and suppurative bacterial infections of the thyroid. These infiltrating infections cause destruction of the thyroid gland and can present with neck pain, thyroid enlargement, and increased thyroxine release. Such patients have initial hyperthyroidism followed by eventual hypothyroidism due to destruction of the gland. Malignancies associated with HIV/AIDS like lymphoma and Kaposi sarcoma have also been rarely reported to infiltrate the thyroid gland and affect its function.

Thyroid Dysfunction in the Immune Reconstitution Inflammatory Syndrome

When a patient with HIV/AIDs is given potent anti-retro viral therapy (ART), autoimmune hypothyroidism may be seen in the setting of improved immunity 3–36 months after the initiation of therapy. The commonly seen condition in this clinical setting is Graves' disease.

Secondary Hypothyroidism

Secondary hypothyroidism has been reported in HIV/AIDS with opportunistic infections affecting the pituitary or the hypothalamus like toxoplasma and CMV. Such patients present with low levels of FT4 with low, inappropriately normal or mildly elevated levels of TSH.

HYPOTHALAMIC-PITUITARY-GONADAL AXIS

Hypogonadism in Males

Hypogonadism can be seen in patients with HIV/AIDS due to multiple reasons. Nearly half of all those infected have biochemical hypogonadism. While secondary hypogonadism is more common, primary hypogonadism is also seen. Whether due to primary or secondary hypogonadism, low testosterone levels are associated with weight loss, progression to AIDS, wasting, depression and loss of muscle mass and exercise capacity.

Secondary Hypogonadism

Malnutrition, which is often seen in the disease, is associated with reduced secretion of gonadotropins by the pituitary. Such down regulation of the hypothalamic-pituitary-gonadal axis (HPG axis) is common to many severe chronic illnesses. Secondly, many opportunistic infections like CMV and *P. jirovecii* can cause destruction of tissues of the pituitary and hypothalamus and cause reduction in the release of gonadotropins. Such patients present with low testosterone levels with low or inappropriately normal levels of luteinizing hormone (LH) and follicle-stimulating hormone (FSH).

Primary Hypogonadism

Primary hypogonadism which presents with a low testosterone level with high gonadotropins occurs more infrequently than secondary hypogonadism. The causes for this are testicular destruction secondary to opportunistic infections like CMV, toxoplasmosis or malignancies like Kaposi sarcoma, and testicular lymphoma.

Drugs also contribute to hypogonadism in HIV/AIDS. Additionally, tumor necrosis factor which is increased in people with HIV/AIDS is known to inhibit testosterone synthesis in the testis.

Drugs Causing Gonadal Dysfunction

The antifungal agent ketoconazole inhibits critical enzymes in testicular steroidogenesis. Megestrol acetate is a synthetic progestational agent that suppresses gonadotropin secretion causing hypogonadism.

INVESTIGATION OF HYPOGONADISM

Free Testosterone versus Total Testosterone

As sex hormone-binding globulin (SHBG) levels are increased to the extent of 55% in patients with HIV/AIDS, it is better to check free testosterone levels rather than total testosterone levels which are artificially high.

Whom to Screen and Whom to Treat?

The Endocrine Society laid out guidelines for testosterone therapy in men with androgen deficiency syndromes in 2010. They suggest testing for testosterone levels in men with symptoms or signs suggestive of hypogonadism which, among others, include reduced muscle bulk and strength often seen in patients with HIV/AIDS.

In the same guidelines, they also recommend short-term testosterone therapy as an adjunctive therapy in HIV-infected men with low testosterone levels and weight loss.

HIV/AIDS and Gonadal Dysfunction in Women

Due to severity of illness and poor nutrition, gonadotropin secretion by the pituitary may be reduced leading to consequent amenorrhea in 25% of women with HIV/AIDS. Other problems that have been reported more commonly among women with HIV /AIDS are anovulation, early menopause and altered menstrual cycles.

Glucose Homeostasis

Infection with HIV has an adverse effect on glucose homeostasis due to both, the disease as well as its treatment. The increased cytokines found in association with the infection are known to increase insulin resistance. Abnormal fat distribution in the form of increased central adiposity and loss of peripheral subcutaneous fat also worsens the insulin resistance. Metabolic abnormalities in HIV have also been shown to be associated with increased levels of retinol binding protein 4 which may further contribute to insulin resistance. Rarely, opportunistic infections destroying the pancreas can lead to reduced beta cell function.

In the era of HAART, the prevalence of disorders of glucose metabolism, including insulin resistance, glucose intolerance and diabetes mellitus has increased due to the effects of anti-retro viral medications. In initial studies in the era of the older anti-retro viral drugs likes tavudine and indinavir, diabetes was found to be 3.1 times more prevalent in HIV-infected people on ART compared to the general population. The advent of newer and safer drugs has reduced, this increased prevalence and some studies have even found that diabetes occurs similarly in HIV-infected and noninfected individuals on newer drugs. What this suggests is that the increased occurrence of diabetes seen with HIV infection may actually be just a consequence of using older ARTs.

The risk factors for developing diabetes in HIV patients have been identified as the drugs patients are treated with and whether or not they develop lipodystrophy. The drugs which are implicated are the older generation drugs like zidovudine, didanosine, lamivudine and stavudine. The role of these drugs in the pathogenesis of diabetes is twofold. Firstly they have a direct adverse effect on glucose metabolism and secondly they contribute to pathogenesis of the disease secondary to increased weight and improvement in diet after initiating therapy.

Lipodystrophy occurs in some patients on ART, especially those onprotease inhibitors. It is characterized by abnormal central fat accumulation (lipohypertrophy) or diffuse loss of fat tissue (lipoatrophy) and is known to predispose the patient toward development of insulin resistance and diabetes.

Among the other drugs, pentamidine which is used for *P. jirovecii* prophylaxis is known to alter glucose metabolism by causing destruction of beta cells of the pancreas.

CONCLUSION

- As the natural history of HIV infection changes due to better healthcare, those infected are living longer and healthier lives. The understanding of the full spectrum of the various opportunistic infections has also increased exponentially over the last couple of decades and affliction of various endocrine organs have been reported to occur with infections by pathogens like CMV, toxoplasma and the tubercular bacilli.
- Knowing about the various endocrine problems which can be expected in a person infected with the HIV virus should help the treating physicians suspect and identify these disorders which often have deceptively innocuous presentations. Though their presenting symptoms and signs may be subtle, endocrinopathies like adrenal insufficiency may have catastrophic consequences if not identified and treated on time.

- While no guidelines exist, universal screening for endocrinopathies is generally not recommended, nor practiced. However, the astute and aware clinician should pick and choose his battles looking for signs and symptoms of hormone excess and deficiencies and test accordingly.
- Additionally, he or she should responsibly marshal his soldiers (drugs in this case) like a good general in a way that they do not harm. It is of utmost importance that while prescribing medicines to treat the primary illness or its complications, we should keep in mind the usual suspects and look for adverse endocrine complications arising out of their use.

"Primum non nocere."

SUGGESTED READING

1. Bhasin S, Cunningham GR, Hayes FJ, et al. Testosterone therapy in men with androgen deficiency syndromes: an Endocrine Society clinical practice guideline. J Clin Endocrinol Metab. 2010;95:2536-5.
2. Bornstein SR, Allolio B, Arlt W, et al. Diagnosis and treatment of primary adrenal insufficiency: An Endocrine Society Clinical Practice Guideline. J Clin Endocrinol Metab. 2016;101:364-89.
3. Brown TT. The effects of HIV-1 infection on endocrine organs. Best Pract Res Clin Endocrinol Metab. 2011;25:403-13.
4. Grinspoon SK. Endocrinology of HIV/AIDS. In: Melmed KS, Polonsky P, Larsen PR, Kronenberg HM (Eds). Williams Textbook of Endocrinology, 13th edition. Philadelphia: Elsiever; 2016. pp. 1776-98.
5. Grinspoon SK, Bilezikian JP. HIV disease and the endocrine system. N Engl J Med. 1992;327:1360-5.
6. Madge S, Smith CJ, Lampe FC, et al. No association between HIV disease and its treatment and thyroid function. HIV Med. 2007;8:22-7.
7. Murphy CS, McKay GA. HIV and diabetes. Diabetes Manage. 2013;3:495-503.
8. Welch K, Finkbeiner W, Alpers CE, et al. Autopsy findings in the acquired immune deficiency syndrome. JAMA. 1984;252:1152-9.

CHAPTER

18

Hematological Manifestations of Human Immunodeficiency Virus Infection

Ajay Sharma

INTRODUCTION

Human immunodeficiency virus (HIV) infection leads to dysregulated immune function, a progressive diminution in the host's immune responses, and an enhanced risk of opportunistic infections. The dysregulated immune function further leads to manifestations such as autoimmune diseases, various organ dysfunction syndromes, and secondary malignancies. Almost any organ system can be involved by HIV infection; the hematological system is primarily involved in almost all patients and is responsible for manifestation of the infection in various forms depending upon the dominant involvement of the bone marrow or peripheral blood.

Although HIV affects the whole immune system, it has a particular propensity for the CD4 surface membrane protein, and results in progressive depletion of helper CD4 thymic lymphocytes with resultant impaired response to soluble antigens, decreased helper response to immunoglobulin synthesis, and impaired delayed hypersensitivity. Also, there is a defective natural killer (NK) function and a decreased T lymphocyte-mediated cytotoxicity of viral infected cells. An imbalance of CD4, CD25, FoxP2+ regulatory cells, and CD4/interleukin (IL)-17 lymphocytes results in the expression of autoreactive T and B lymphocytes. This leads to an increased incidence of autoimmune disorders associated with HIV infection.

CD4 DEPLETION

The hallmark of HIV infection is CD4+ lymphopenia. It is responsible for various complications of the disease. The CD4 depletion occurs due to various mechanisms in the HIV infection. The most prominent cause of CD4 depletion is by a direct cytopathic effect on replication of CD4 lymphocytes. In addition, the infected CD4 cells, through gp120, fuse with uninfected CD4 cells, and thus result in further depletion of CD4 helper cells. CD4 cells are also depleted due to the host reaction against the virus. The CD4 cells are also destroyed by an "innocent bystander" mechanism secondary to binding of the free gp120 to their surface CD4 protein.

Although CD4+ lymphopenia dominates the clinical spectrum, approximately 50% patients develop neutropenia, reflecting the non-T-cell myelosuppressive effect of HIV infection. In addition, anemia occurs in 70–80% of patients with HIV infection and 40–50% patients develop thrombocytopenia during active HIV infection.

Human immunodeficiency virus infection also results in depletion of myeloid and erythroid colony forming precursor activity. This is due to an indirect rather than to a direct effect on the CD4+ cells. Since, stem cells (CD34+ cells) lack CD4, and other infection facilitating proteins, viz. CXCR4 and CCR5, they are not infected by HIV. The replication of the virus in the bone marrow microenvironment is essential for decreased hematopoietic cell production during HIV infection.

Mononuclear macrophage cells, once infected by HIV release aberrant cytokines like transforming growth factor-β (TGF-β), tumor necrosis factor-α (TNF-α), and IL-1 with resultant suppression of hematopoiesis. TNF-α is a potent mediator of inflammation and host response to the infectious process. It results in tissue damage, muscle wasting impaired hematopoiesis's suppressive effect of viral replication on hematopoiesis is highlighted by the fact that with initiation of highly active anti-retro viral therapy (HAART), resulting in a decrease in viral load leads to restoration of hematopoiesis in the patient.

Human immunodeficiency virus infection can present with one of the hematological manifestations before being diagnosed, or the course of the disease may be complicated by one or more manifestations of an hematological nature (Table 18.1). A thorough understanding of the pathophysiology of such disorders helps in optimal management of a patient with HIV infection.

ANEMIA

Anemia is the most frequent cytopenia encountered in HIV-1 infection. Severe anemia requiring frequent transfusions was seen more often during the early years if the epidemic when Zidovudine was used in most of the patients. With the advent of newer drugs, the incidence of severe anemia has decreased significantly. But it may still be seen in advanced chronic disease. Persistent anemia is associated with short survival, independent of the degree of immunosuppression. Anemia results due to one of the four major factors:

1. Ineffective erythropoiesis
2. Red blood cell (RBC) destruction
3. Blood loss due to invasive infections of the intestine [cytomegalovirus (CMV) or Kaposi's sarcoma (KS)]

Table 18.1: Hematological manifestations of human immunodeficiency virus infection.

1	*Unexplained anemia:* ▪ Nutritional anemia ▪ Immune hemolytic anemia ▪ Hemolytic anemia due to drugs used in HAART ▪ Refractory anemia due to HIV infection induced bone marrow dysplasia ▪ *Microangiopathy hemolytic anemia (MHA):* • Disseminated intravascular coagulation (DIC) • Thrombotic thrombocytopenic purpura (TTP)
2	*Bone marrow failure:* ▪ *Bone marrow aplasia:* Secondary aplastic anemia ▪ *Isolated cytopenia:* • Thrombocytopenia • Neutropenia • Agranulocytosis
3	*Immune cytopenia:* ▪ Immune-mediated thrombocytopenia ▪ Immune-mediated pancytopenia
4	*HIV-associated lymphomas:* ▪ *Lymphomas that occur with reasonable frequency:* • Burkitt lymphoma • Diffuse large B-cell lymphoma • Extranodal marginal zone B-cell lymphoma of mucosa associated lymphoid tissue (MALT) • Peripheral T-cell lymphoma • Classic Hodgkin's lymphoma. ▪ Unusual lymphoma occurring more specifically in HIC infection.

(HAART: Highly active anti-retro viral therapy; HIV: Human immunodeficiency virus).

4. Decreased red cell production due to HIV infection, cytokines interfering with hematopoiesis, HAART, and medications used to treat the opportunistic infections, including high-dose Trimethoprim-sulfamethoxazole (TMP/SMX) for *Pneumocystis carinii* for pneumonia and Ganciclovir for CMV infection. This may also be seen due to bone marrow infiltration by HIV-associated lymphoma, low erythropoietin

Impact of Anemia on Human Immunodeficiency Virus Disease

The severity of anemia correlates with the disease progression and has a direct impact on the mortality. The virus may also have a direct effect on erythropoiesis. This has been shown by the resolution of anemia with HAART. It has been identified as an independent prognostic marker in HIV patients. It has also been associated with shortened median survival irrespective of their initial CD4+ count. Anemia as well as CD4 counts are known to be independent prognostic factors associated with mortality.

What Causes Anemia in Human Immunodeficiency Virus Infection?

Anemia can occur either due to decreased production or increased destruction. The most common cause of anemia in HIV disease is decreased RBC production (Table 18.2). Frequently encountered mechanisms responsible for decreased RBC production include the anemia of acute and chronic inflammation, infection, or infiltration of bone marrow by infective agents, viz. atypical mycobacteria, tuberculosis, cytomegalovirus, fungal infections, etc. Malignancies too can involve marrow as in the case of lymphoma and KS. Parvovirus B19 can cause isolated pure red cell aplasia in severely immunocompromised patients. Medications used in treatment or prophylaxis can also result in bone marrow suppression. Nutritional deficiencies, viz. B12/folate result in ineffective hematopoiesis.

Other causes of anemia include anemia secondary to blood loss or hemolysis. The latter is due to drugs, glucose-6-phosphate dehydrogenase (G6PD) deficiency, thrombotic thrombocytopenic purpura, hemophagocytic syndrome, viral infections, and organ damage like liver dysfunction, chronic renal disease, etc.

<table>
<tr><th colspan="2">Table 18.2: Causes of anemia in human immunodeficiency virus (HIV).</th></tr>
<tr><td>1</td><td>HIV related:
▪ HIV virus related:
• Blunted production/response to erythropoietin
• Anemia of chronic disease
• Suppression of CFU-GEMM (through inflammatory cytokines)
▪ Bone marrow infection:
• Parvovirus B19
• Mycobacterium tuberculosis
• Atypical Mycobacterium
• Histoplasma
• Cytomegalovirus
▪ Malignancies infiltrating bone marrow:
• Non-Hodgkin's lymphoma
• Kaposi sarcoma
• Hodgkin's lymphoma</td></tr>
<tr><td>2</td><td>Medications<table><tr><th>Decreased production</th><th>Hemolysis</th></tr><tr><td>▪ Reverse transcriptase inhibitors
▪ Ganciclovir
▪ Bactrim
▪ Amphotericin-B</td><td>▪ Indinavir
▪ Dapsone
▪ Bactrim
▪ Antibiotics</td></tr></table></td></tr>
<tr><td>3</td><td>HIV unrelated:
▪ B12/folic acid deficiency
▪ Iron deficiency (malabsorption/blood loss)</td></tr>
</table>

Therapy

The treatment of anemia should be directed toward correcting the underlying cause whenever feasible. The use of blood transfusion should be minimized and reserved for patients with symptomatic anemia, extremely low hemoglobin (Hb) levels, and a rapidly falling Hb. The use of HAART has shown that suppression of HIV replication itself is associated with improvement in the Hb level. This improvement is independent of changes in the CD4+ lymphocyte count. The improvement can be noticed as early as 8–12 weeks, with maximal improvement obtained usually by 12 months. The combination therapies may sometimes have to be used, when a critically sick patient's condition does not permit a detailed time-consuming workup looking for the cause of anemia.

Erythropoietin use has been shown to be a useful modality of therapy in chronic anemia, when all treatable causes have been excluded. A blunted response to EPO, as observed in the anemia of acute and chronic inflammation, is common in HIV infection. But the use of EPO for anemia should be restricted to symptomatic patients with Hb levels less than expected for their age and sex. The initial adult dose is 40,000 units subcutaneously weekly or 100–200 units/kg three times per week. The onset of action can take 2–6 weeks, while an increase in reticulocyte count can be seen within 1–2 weeks. The baseline level of endogenous serum EPO has been shown to be predictive of the response to the therapeutic use of EPO with a baseline level of more than 500 IU/L being associated with a low response to treatment. Response to EPO may also depend upon the severity of the anemia, presence of active infection, inflammation, and available iron stores. Hence, a comprehensive approach may be required rather than empirical therapy with hematinics. The combination of EPO therapy, cART, and specific targeted therapy may yield the best and prompt response in a case of refractory to initial therapy.

CYTOPENIA IN HUMAN IMMUNODEFICIENCY VIRUS INFECTION

Cytopenia is common in patients with advanced HIV infection. Low white cell counts are frequently a result of both decreased lymphocytes as well as neutrophils. The risk factors for neutropenia include a high level of plasma HIV, viral ribonucleic acid (RNA), and a low CD4+ lymphocyte count. The use of HAART is associated with a lower risk for developing neutropenia. The decrease in the neutrophil count is often transient, self limiting, and rarely of clinical significance, but a neutrophil count of less than 500/cm^2 of prolonged duration does pose a significant risk for infection. The most common cause for such a low count is drug-related myelosuppression or overwhelming superinfection by opportunistic or other organisms. The neutropenia often improves with control of infections and HAART administration, the neutropenia related to drugs like Zidovudine can continue, and may necessitate a change in therapy. It is rare, but agranulocytosis does occur with anti-retro viral drugs like abacavir and indinavir. A number of acquired functional defects have been described in both neutrophils and monocytes from patients with HIV infection. Many of these defects are observed in patients with advanced disease with high viral load and severe CD4+ lymphopenia.

The treatment of neutropenia is often a problem. The underlying cause should be treated. This may entail altering the drug therapy and aggressive treatment of resistant infections. The granulocyte-macrophage colony-stimulating factors (GM-CSFs) or granulocyte colony stimulating factors (G-CSFs) are the primary pharmacological agents used in the treatment of severe HIV-related neutropenia and have been found to be safe and effective. They should be only used if the absolute neutrophil count (ANC) is less than $500/cm^2$ and accompanied by bone pains and headache. Its common side effects are fever, myalgia, and fatigue.

HUMAN IMMUNODEFICIENCY VIRUS INFECTION AND LYMPHOMA

The spectrum of lymphoproliferative diseases in HIV infections is wide and varied (Table 18.1). 10–15% of patients with HIV infection will develop non-Hodgkin's lymphoma (NHL). The incidence of lymphomas, especially of the B-cell type, has been seen to be more common in immunocompromised individuals, whether it is due to the immunodeficiency produced by the virus, the virus itself, or the drug-related immunosuppression, as well as post transplant immunosuppressive therapy. After the advent of HAART, the incidence of HIV associated B-cell lymphoma has decreased markedly. In addition, the host biology might also contribute toward the lymphoma tumor genesis.

Although KS, aggressive B-cell lymphoma and cervical cancers are said to be acquired immunodeficiency syndrome (AIDS) defining when they occurring in the setting of HIV infection, death from non-AIDS defining cancers is more common. The development of malignancies can be related to factors like concurrent infections with viruses like the human herpesvirus-8 (HHV-8), and Epstein-Barr virus (EBV), or human papillomavirus, which foster malignant transformation. The viruses carry oncogenic proteins and cytokines that contribute to malignancy. Additionally, HIV infection reduces the ability to clear the viral infection. Even disruptions in HAART can increase the risk significantly. Although the incidence of KS and other certain lymphomas has decreased after HAART was introduced, the frequency of other tumors such as cervical cancer has remained unchanged. Central nervous system (CNS) lymphoma, once accounting for 18% of AIDS-related

Table 18.3: WHO-based classification of HIV-associated lymphomas.	
1	*Lymphomas which occur with reasonable frequency in the absence of HIV infection:* ▪ Burkitt lymphoma ▪ Diffuse large B-cell lymphoma • Centroblastic lymphoma • Immunoblastic lymphoma ▪ Extranodal marginal zone B-cell lymphoma of the mucosa associated lymphoid tissue ▪ Peripheral T-cell lymphoma ▪ Classic Hodgkin's lymphoma
2	*Unusual lymphoma, occurring more specifically in HIV infection:* ▪ Primary effusion lymphoma ▪ Plasmablastic lymphoma
3	*Lymphomas occurring in other immune deficiency states:* ▪ Polymorphic B-cell lymphoma

(HIV: Human immunodeficiency virus; WHO: World Health Organization).

lymphomas, is now quite rare. The improved drug therapies for lymphomas as well as the availability of HAART have contributed to improvements in morbidity and mortality.

Non-Hodgkin's lymphoma and Hodgkin's lymphoma (HL) occur more frequently in patients with HIV infection. Approximately 10% of HIV-positive patients will develop NHL. Although, the incidence has greatly been reduced after HAART, it is still 25–150-fold higher than seen in a non-HIV population. Decreased immune surveillance, B-cell dysregulation, and in some cases, infection with HHV-8 and EBV are also involved in the pathophysiology of the disorder. With HAART, the incidence of lymphomas associated with low CD4+ counts has been reduced significantly, but NHL occurring at higher CD4 counts has been relatively been unaffected. Three types of lymphoma are now recognized as AIDS defining by the Centers for Disease Control and Prevention (CDC) in the United States of America. These include:

1. Burkitt's lymphoma.
2. Immunoblastic lymphoma, a subtype of diffuse large B-cell lymphoma (DLBCL)
3. Primary CNS lymphoma (Table 18.3).

Among patients with systemic AIDS-related NHL, there has been decreased high-grade histology and improved survival. But still, 70–90% of AIDS-related lymphomas are highly aggressive and are almost exclusively the immunoblastic variant of DLBCL and Burkitt's lymphoma. T-cell lymphomas are uncommon in HIV disease. Still, the incidence of such lymphomas is 15-fold higher in HIV-positive population compared with general population. The indolent lymphomas are also uncommon, comprising less than 10% of AIDS-related lymphomas.

Risk Factors for Lymphomas in Human Immunodeficiency Virus

Risk factors for AIDS-related lymphoma include both HIV-specific factors (CD4 count, HIV viral load) as well as more general risk factors known to increase the risk of NHL in such patients. These include low CD4 count, HIV viral load, early HAART institution (this has decreased the incidence of NHL), and B-cell abnormalities indicating the B-cell activation, e.g. high total serum immunoglobulins, detectable serum soluble CD30, and elevated serum free light chain levels increase the risk for NHL. Other risk factors include genetic predisposition (CCR5-32 deletion with a higher risk) and family history.

Therapy

The outcome of therapy has greatly improved after the adoption of HAART in the management. Prior to the HAART era, most protocols used truncated combination therapies with inferior results with shorter durations of remission and survival of the patients with lymphoma used to be dismal. With HAART, the CD4 counts improved and more intensive therapies could be used. The HAART therapy itself has induced remission occasionally, but it is not the standard of care and most trials now focus on more intensive therapies.

The therapies are tailored according to the level of preexisting immunosuppression, with low versus high-dose therapies in patients with moderate and severe immunosuppression. Patients with CD4 counts over 0.2×10^9/L receive dose-intensified regimens, including the well-known protocol "CHOP" in modified doses (Cyclophosphamide, Doxorubicin, Vincristine, and Prednisolone) with or without Rituximab. The results of low-dose CHOP have been compared with standard dose schedules and the results have been found to be same, provided the CD4 counts are above 0.2×10^9/L. A number of other combination therapies have been used with variable results. They include EPOCH (Etoposide, Prednisolone, Vincristine, Cyclophosphamide, and Doxorubicin-Cyclophosphamide dose adjusted to CD4 counts). Such modifications have produced remission responses in approximately 80% of patients.

Burkitt's lymphoma, which is highly overrepresented in patients living with HIV, has had a poor outcome due to prolonged neutropenia with standard therapies. A prospective AIDS Malignancy Consortium-048 (AMC-048) study has shown promising results with modifications in protocols like CODOX-M/IVAC, indicating that standard CHOP therapy may not be a best option in Burkitt's lymphoma.

Hodgkin's Lymphoma

Even though it is not considered to be an AIDS defining illness, a marked increase in its incidence is seen in HIV. HL is among the most common non-AIDS defining malignancies, with an incidence of 15–30-fold higher than in the non-HIV population. Unlike HL in HIV-uninfected patients, B symptoms are almost often present. Unfavorable histology is more common with mixed cellularity accounting for 60% of patients and advanced (in 70–80% of cases), extranodal disease is mostly seen (>60% cases) in these patients. Unlike those not infected with HIV, noncontiguous spread of disease is common and mediastinal involvement is less common. Bone marrow involvement is almost invariably present. Another feature distinguishing HIV-associated HL is the predominance of Reed–Sternberg cell rich cases. Most of these patients are EBV positive. The pathological role of EBV in HL is evidenced by the Reed-Sternberg cell expression of EBV transforming protein. There is no evidence of definitive correlation of CD4 count with the incidence of HL.

Hodgkin's Lymphoma Therapy

The standard combination therapy with ABVD (doxorubicin, bleomycin, vinblastine, and dacarbazine) protocol has not been shown to show the optimal results. But with HAART therapy, its results are likely to be much better. Recent studies in the HAART era have shown a better outcome with addition of biological therapies like addition of anti-CD30 antibody (Brentuximab vedotin).

Hematopoietic Stem Cell Transplantation in HIV-associated Lymphoma

Before the advent of HAART, the median survival for relapsed HIV-related NHL with standard chemotherapy was less than 1 year and even with HAART, the outcome in a relapsed patient is likely to be poor so the need for alternate approach is important. There have been a few studies with a small number of patients undergoing transplants which have shown that outcome can be improved with the appropriate use of HAART, so that once a patient achieves a state of CD4 count less than 10,000 cells/mm^3 by reverse transcriptase polymerase chain reaction (RT-PCR). The 3-year progression free survival (PFS) was 76%. Another study by an Italian group reported similar results. Allogeneic transplants have been attempted with a nonmyeloablative approach, but so far, the results are not very promising in this group of patients. Overall, autologous transplant is a viable option in a relapsed patient, who has received HAART, has a good performance status (>2), has an uninvolved bone marrow, and has a CD count less than 100 cells/μL.

HUMAN IMMUNODEFICIENCY VIRUS RESERVOIR

It has been shown that HIV-1 can be isolated from the blood of patients on HAART, when HIV-1 RNA levels are undetectable by the most sensitive tools. This suggests that there could be one or more sanctuary sites which are resistant to best form of therapies, and can be responsible for recurrence of infection. Thes etheoretical sites are believed to consist of CD4+ lymphocytes and dendritic cells. The latter, can specifically be responsible for the relapse of infection. Whether autologous stem cell transplantation, wherein the patient's own cells might be reinfused, would offer a long-term survival benefit will be a moot question. The role of allogeneic stem cell transplantation in this context also needs to be defined.

CONCLUSION

- Human immunodeficiency virus infection is fast changing in its natural history after the advent of HAART. The patient's with HIV infections are living longer, and are at the threshold of getting cured. The incidence of opportunistic infection is on the decline. Their life expectancy could approach that of the general population.
- Cytopenia, particularly anemia, is more common in the advanced stages of the disease and results both from bone marrow failure and peripheral destruction. While HAART has turned the tide highly in favor of improving outcomes, two complications are getting highlighted at this stage.
- The increasing morbidity due to the drug (used during the treatment of these patients) toxicities and increasing mortality due to AIDS defining as well as non-AIDS defining malignancies.
- Lymphomas are highly prevalent among the HIV-infected population, although CNS lymphoma has become quite rare after HAART.
- The encouraging fact is that with HAART, intensive combination chemotherapies can now be used more effectively, with the prospect of achieving long-term remissions. The possibility of improvements in long-term survival has further been reinforced by the availability of specific monoclonal antibodies like anti-CD30 antibody conjugated to an antitubulin drug (Brentuximab vedotin).
- In future, it is likely that the focus will shift toward prevention of inciting viral infections like EBV and HHV-8. Another step will be to achieve immune reconstitution, rather than just a chemotherapy-based approach. This will go a long way toward improving survival and achieving clinically significant cure rates.

SUGGESTED READING

1. Hoffman DM, Caruso RF, Mirando T. Human immunodeficiency virus-associated thrombocytopenia. DICP. 1989;23(2):157-60.

2. Levy R, Colonna P, Tourani JM, et al. Human immunodeficiency virus associated Hodgkin's disease: report of 45 cases from the French Registry of HIV-Associated Tumors. Leukemia & Lymphoma. 1995;16(5-6):451-6.
3. Mehta S, Jutur S, Gautam D. Hematologic manifestations of HIV/AIDS. Medicine Update. 2011;9:484-90.
4. Opie J. Haematological complications of HIV infection. South African Medical Journal. 2012;102(6):465-8.
5. Parinitha SS, Kulkarni MH. Haematological changes in HIV infection with correlation to CD4 cell count. Australas Med J. 2012;5(3):157.

CHAPTER 19

Skin Manifestations in HIV

Divya Arora, Shilpa Garg

INTRODUCTION

Skin is a common organ which is involved in patients with people living with HIV/AIDS (PLHA). Many a time the diagnosis of HIV is made by initial skin involvement. The overview of skin manifestation in HIV is given below.

STAGES OF HIV AND SKIN INVOLVEMENT

The human immunodeficiency virus (HIV) is a retrovirus and is mainly of two types—HIV-1 and HIV-2 with HIV-1 being mainly responsible for the worldwide pandemic. The history of HIV infection dates back to 1981, when the Centers for Disease Control and Prevention (CDC) in the United States of America noticed the occurrence of uncommon infections like *Pneumocystis carinii* pneumonia, in clusters. This led to a diagnosis of an acquired immunodeficiency syndrome (AIDS). Ever since then, the number of HIV-infected people has been on a rise, irrespective of geographical barriers. Sexual intercourse, blood transfusion and vertical transmission from mother to baby are the common modes of acquiring the infection.

The natural history of HIV infection has been classified by the World Health Organization (WHO) into acute primary infection followed by four stages.

Acute primary infection: Symptoms of an acute HIV infection are mild and commonly include fever, rash, fatigue, pharyngitis, weight loss, night sweats, lymphadenopathy, myalgias, headache, nausea, and diarrhea. The skin may show erythematous flat (macules) or elevated (papules) lesions, distributed all over the body including the palms and soles. It may be associated with oral and genital ulceration.

Stage 1: The patient mostly remains asymptomatic at this stage. Lymph node palpation may reveal persistent generalized lymphadenopathy.

Stage 2: As the disease progresses, the patient may have weight loss which is less than 10% of the normal weight. Herpes zoster, fungal infections, and angular cheilitis are common skin manifestations. The patient may also complain of nonspecific itchy eruptions on the body. There may be a history of exacerbation of pre-existing dermatoses like dandruff and itchiness on the scalp.

Stage 3: The patient becomes more debilitated at stage 3 which is characterized by a weight loss of more than 10% of the pre-existing weight or has persistent diarrhea or fever lasting more than a month. There is a flare up of multiple infections like reactivation of pulmonary tuberculosis or severe respiratory tract infections.

The oral mucosa shows persistent white plaques which can be scraped off easily suggestive of candidiasis. Also commonly seen is oral hairy leukoplakia which is characterized by a white corrugated plaque on the lateral aspect of the tongue.

Stage 4: This stage, also known as the HIV wasting syndrome, is characterized by recurrent herpes simplex infection, disseminated cutaneous tuberculosis, cryptococcosis, histoplasmosis and a number of atypical infections not commonly seen in an immunocompetent host.

While the characteristic pattern of skin changes in each stage may give a hint to the diagnosis, cutaneous dermatosis in an HIV-positive patient can also be classified into infective and noninfective.

INFECTIVE DERMATOSES

Viral Infections

In an HIV-infected patient, not only are viral infections more common, they are also more severe.

Herpes simplex virus (HSV) infection is characterized by multiple fluid-filled lesions at the angles of the mouth or on the genitals. In a seropositive patient, the vesicles may be multiple, rupture to form deep ulcers and may extend over a larger surface area like the buccal mucosa, tongue and palate in HSV-1 infection and buttocks and perineum in HSV-2 (Fig. 19.1). Antiviral medications like acyclovir 400 mg three times a day need to be given for 10 days to 2 weeks.

Herpes zoster infection presents usually with grouped vesicles in the distribution of a single dermatome. However, in an immunocompromised host, it may be multidermatomal, and lead to the formation of large ulcers or heal with extensive scarring (Fig. 19.2). Such patients need to be treated aggressively with acyclovir tablets 800 mg five times a day for 10 days or more. In disseminated, visceral, or eye involvement with herpes zoster, acyclovir 10 mg/kg/body weight intravenously every 8 hours is given for 7 days.

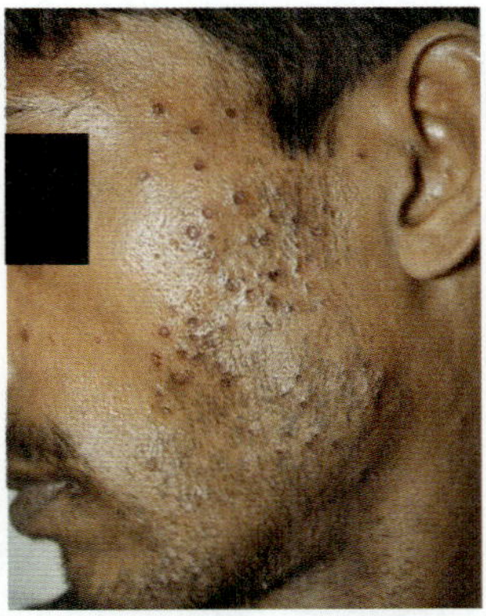

Fig. 19.1: Herpes simplex—primary infection with lesions involving the entire cheek.

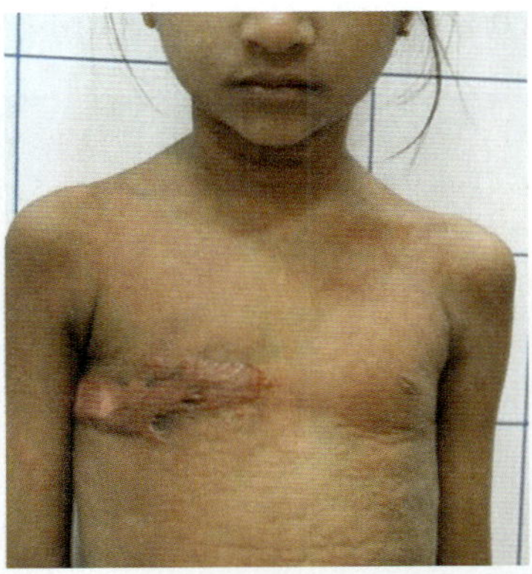

Fig. 19.2: Keloid at the site of herpes zoster in an HIV-positive young girl. Note the maculopapular drug rash on the body after starting nevirapine-based ART.

Infections like *molluscum contagiosum* characterized by asymptomatic small pearly white papules in a healthy host, may be more numerous and bigger in size (Fig. 19.3). They are generally more resistant to treatment. Electrofulguration may be required besides needling of the molluscum.

Likewise, warts caused by *human papillomavirus* (HPV) may be more widespread and confluent and resistant to treatment. Frequency of other viral infections like oral hairy leukoplakia caused by the Epstein-Barr virus and cytomegalovirus infections also increases.

Bacterial Infections

A common boil also known as *folliculitis* is the most common bacterial infection seen in HIV-positive patients. The rates of *Staphylococcus aureus* infection are much higher in these patients leading to folliculitis, furuncles and impetigo which is characterized by a honey-colored crust predominantly seen on the face.

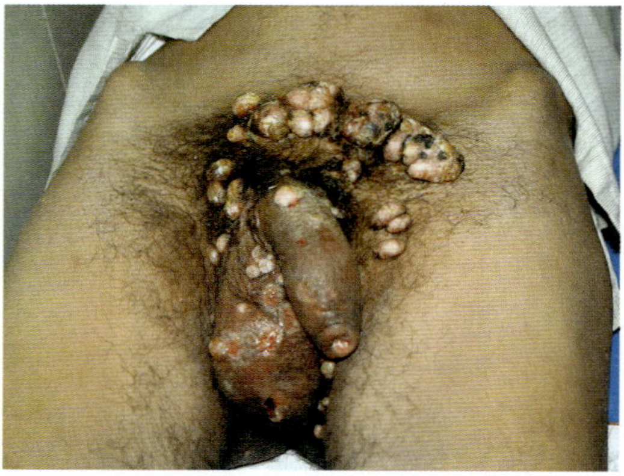

Fig. 19.3: Giant molluscum with secondary infection on the suprapubic area, groin and scrotum. Patient had coexisting herpes genitalis lesions.

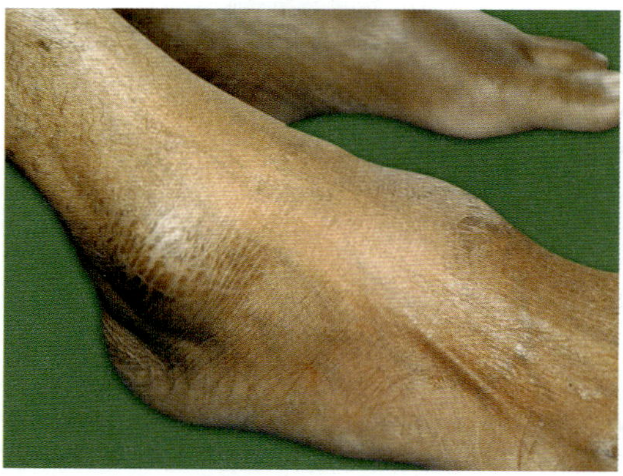

Fig. 19.4: Asymptomatic soft swelling over the ankle in an immunocompromised patient. Staining of the aspirate revealed acid-fast bacilli.

Reactivation or reinfection of *Mycobacterium tuberculosis* is seen in a number of patients. A large nonhealing painless ulcer overlying a lymph node may suggest scrofuloderma. Multiple fluid-filled abscesses which are red to violaceous and painless, in a debilitated patient, are likely to be metastatic tubercular gummata, a disseminated form of cutaneous tuberculosis (Fig. 19.4). Antitubercular therapy consisting of four drugs namely rifampicin, isoniazid, pyrazinamide and ethionamide, for a minimum duration of 6 months is the treatment of choice.

Atypical mycobacterial infections like *Mycobacterium avium-intracellulare* are also more common in immunocompromised hosts.

Pseudomonal infection of the skin and nails is seen more frequently in these patients.

Bacillary angiomatosis is a bacterial disease caused by the Gram-negative organism *Bartonella henselae*. Patient presents with red flesh-colored papules on the skin or mucous membrane. These lesions need to be differentiated from Kaposi's sarcoma as they are treatable with erythromycin 2 g/day or doxycycline for 3–4 weeks which is sufficient to clear the infection.

Fungal Infections

Superficial and deep fungal infections are more common and more widespread in a seropositive patient.

Dermatophyte infections namely tinea cruris, tinea corporis, onychomycosis, and tinea capitis involve a large surface area compared to a healthy host. In a severely immunocompromised individual, the typical central clearing and elevated margins may not be seen. They are more resistant to treatment and antifungals like itraconazole 100 mg twice daily need to be given for 2–4 weeks.

Candidiasis caused by the yeast *Candida albicans*, is an important marker of HIV infection and can manifest in varied forms. At one end of the spectrum is oropharyngeal candidiasis seen clinically as a creamy white plaque in the oral cavity which can be easily scraped off. It is an early marker of HIV infection. Esophageal candidiasis is an indicator of disease progression. At the other end of the spectrum is disseminated candidiasis which presents with papules and pustules all over the body.

Vulvovaginal candidiasis and candidal nail infection may be other manifestations of the disease in an HIV-positive patient. Fluconazole 150 mg for 7–14 days is the treatment of choice.

Deep fungal infections like cryptococcosis, histoplasmosis and penicilliosis are seen when the CD4 cell count falls below 100. Cryptococcosis presents with molluscum-like lesions, i.e. papules with a central umbilication. A high degree of clinical suspicion is therefore required. Demonstration of the capsulated organism on India ink staining confirms the diagnosis.

Parasitic Infections

Scabies caused by the mite *Sarcoptes scabiei*, is a common parasitic infestation in HIV patients. Like candidiasis, the extent of the disease is suggestive of the immune status of patient. Norwegian scabies is the severe variety characterized by colonization of the skin by millions of mites. The patient presents in erythroderma with thick crusted plaques all over the body. Oral ivermectinis the treatment of choice and multiple applications of 5% permethrin may be required to clear the infection.

Demodex folliculorum is a mite which is normally present on facial skin. However, in an HIV patient as the immunity goes down, it presents with multiple itchy papules and nodules on the eyelids, face, and neck. It responds well to oral ivermectin.

NONINFECTIVE DERMATOSES

The cutaneous features in case of an HIV patient which are not related to skin infections can be divided into those arising as a part of the disease complex and those arising secondary to treatment.

Inflammatory diseases of the skin like psoriasis, reactive arthritis and seborrheic dermatitis are usually more extensive than in non-HIV patients.

A patient with psoriasis may directly present at a stage when his entire body is involved, i.e. in erythroderma. Careful examination of the skin, hair and nails may give a clue to the diagnosis.

Seborrheic dermatitis presenting with thick greasy scales involving the scalp, eyebrows, eyelids and neck, is more common, even in presence of a high CD4 count. Extensive presentation in a previously healthy individual is, in fact, considered to be an early marker of HIV. Oral fluconazole and ketoconazole salicylic acid-based washes are useful. Starting antiretroviral therapy (ART) itself may be curative in some patients.

Another set of cutaneous disorders typically seen in HIV patients is the development of itchy papules and pustules on the upper body in case of *eosinophilic folliculitis* and predominantly on the extensors in case of *papular pruritic eruptions*. The patient needs to be treated with oral prednisolone in case of eosinophilic folliculitis whereas antihistamines and topical steroids usually suffice in the latter group.

Skin malignancies like Kaposi's sarcoma also occur in higher frequency in AIDS patients. They present with bluish vascular nodules in the oral cavity or on the skin. Early treatment with ART may control disease progression.

Patients who have been started on oral ART may show different cutaneous features. Zidovudine therapy gives rise to bluish gray discoloration of the nails and elongation of the eyelashes. Gray nails may be an indicator of decreased CD4 count.

A physician should be on a watch for signs of drug reaction once ART is started. They range from red maculopapular rashes involving the entire body to widespread bulla formation including the eyes and oral and genital mucosa (Fig. 19.5). Non-nucleoside reverse transcriptase inhibitors (NNRTIs) like nevirapine, delavirdine, and efavirenz; the nucleoside reverse transcriptase inhibitors (NRTIs) like abacavir, and the protease inhibitor (PI) like amprenavir are the drugs commonly implicated in the development of severe adverse drug reactions.

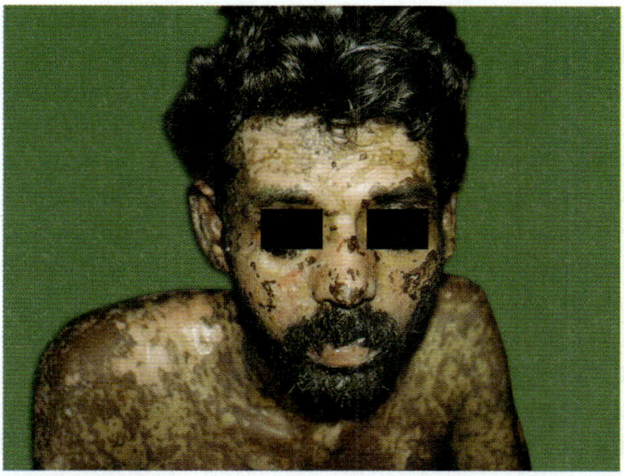

Fig. 19.5: Patient with toxic epidermal necrolysis 2 weeks after starting ART.

The offending agent needs to be identified and stopped immediately.

Lastly certain dermatoses may downgrade after starting ART. Immune reconstitution inflammatory syndrome is the term used for paradoxical worsening of pre-existing skin diseases probably secondary to the recovery of immune status. Cutaneous tuberculosis, herpes zoster, cutaneous warts, urticarial hives may be seen within 2 months of starting HIV medications. These should be treated as per their respective guidelines and ART should be continued.

CONCLUSION

The skin being the body's largest organ, reflects the underlying immune status of a patient in different forms. It helps not only in diagnosis but also in predicting the prognosis of an infected patient. A careful eye and an educated mind can lead to the early diagnosis and successful management of multiple diseases in an immune susceptible host. It goes a long way in decreasing the morbidity and improving the quality of life in such patients.

SUGGESTED READING

1. Boonchai W, Laohasrisakul R, Manonukul J, et al. Pruritic papular eruption in HIV seropositive patients: a cutaneous marker for immunosuppression. Int J Dermatol. 1999;38(5):348-50.
2. Crum-Cianflone N, Hullsiek KH, Satter E, et al. Cutaneous malignancies among HIV-infected persons. Arch Intern Med. 2009;169(12):1130-8.
3. Dharmshale SN, Patil SA, Gohil A, et al. Disseminated crytococcosis with extensive cutaneous involvement in AIDS. Indian J Med Microbiol. 2006;24(3):228-30.
4. High WA, Evans CC, Hoang MP. Cutaneous miliary tuberculosis in two patients with HIV infection.J Am Acad Dermatol. 2004;50(5 Suppl):S110-3.
5. Janniger CK, Gascon P, Schwartz RA, et al. Erythroderma as the initial presentation of the acquired immunodeficiency syndrome. Dermatologica. 1991;183(2):143-5.

6. Kar HK, Narayan R, Gautam RK, et al. Mucocutaneous disorders in HIV positive patients. Indian J Dermatol Venereol Leprol. 1996;62:283-5.
7. Plettenberg A, Lorenzen T, Burtsche BT, et al. Bacillary angiomatosis in HIV-infected patients—an epidemiological and clinical study. Dermatology. 2000;201(4):326-31.
8. Rex JH, Walsh TJ, Sobel JD, et al. Practice guidelines for the treatment of candidiasis. Infectious Diseases Society of America. Clin Infect Dis. 2000;30:662-78.
9. Saka B, Barro-Traore F, Atadokpede FA, et al. Stevens-Johnson syndrome and toxic epidermal necrolysis in sub-Saharan Africa: a multicentric study in four countries. Int J Dermatol. 2013;52(5):575-9.
10. Sentamilselvi G, Janaki C, Ajithandas K, et al. Chronic dermatophytosis. Indian J Dermatol. 2000;45:168-73.
11. Severson JL, Tyring SK. Relation between herpes simplex viruses and human immunodeficiency virus infections. Arch Dermatol. 1999;135:1393-7.
12. Singh A, Thappa DM, Hamide A. The spectrum of mucocutaneous manifestations during the evolutionary phases of HIV disease: an emerging Indian scenario. J Dermatol (Tokyo). 1999;26:294-304.
13. Wiederkehr M, Schwartz RA. Giant proliferative molluscumcontagiosum. Acta Derm Venereol (Ljubljana). 2002;11:101-4.
14. Zampogna JC, Flowers FP. Persistent verrucous varicella as the initial manifestation of HIV infection. J Am Acad Dermatol. 2001;44(2 Suppl):391-4.

CHAPTER

20

Bone Health in HIV/AIDS

Atul Kakar

INTRODUCTION

As the life-expectancy of people living with HIV/AIDS (PLHA) increases, many metabolic issues have emerged, including the loss of bone mineral density (BMD). In many subjects, this leads to osteopenia or osteoporosis. The awareness of bone health is lacking and is not a priority for physicians who are treating PLHA. Vitamin-D deficiency is rampant in India and is a major risk factor contributing toward low bone density in PLHA. Although HIV per se contributes toward the incidence of osteopenia/osteoporosis, other risk factors like drugs (e.g. Tenofovir), smoking, substance abuse may also add to this problem.

EFFECT OF HIV ON BONES

A review of recent data shows that there is an increase in the prevalence of low bone mineral density in PLHA. The onset of menopause causes osteopenia/osteoporosis within a few years and similar changes result from HIV virus infection and after the initiation of anti-retro viral therapy. Recent studies have also suggested an increase in fracture rates in the HIV-infected population. Many of these fractures can be prevented if physicians are aware about bone health issues. In a meta-analysis, the prevalence of osteoporosis was three times higher among HIV infected subjects than those who were HIV negative especially if they were receiving anti-retro viral therapy.

Osteoporosis has a devastating effect on the entire skeleton. This disease causes fractures which increases healthcare costs to patients and to society. The two important sites of fractures are the vertebrae and hip. Both these may have serious consequences on a patient's health—whereas former causes severe back pain and deformity the latter may lead tolong term and permanent disability or require a major surgical procedure which carries a certain mortality.

RISK FACTORS

There are many factors which can cause low BMD in patients with HIV infection. There is a complex interaction between HIV infection, traditional osteoporosis risk factors and those which are related to anti-retro viral treatment. The effect of poor nutrition due to chronic HIV infection and low weight, smoking, substance use, alcohol abuse, hypovitaminosis D, and ART use can further exacerbate bone loss. ART-naive patients also have a high prevalence of low bone density, which is due to uncontrolled HIV. The viremia can cause systemic inflammation which in turn can have an effect on bone remodeling. HIV proteins cause an imbalance between the osteoblastic and osteoclastic activities of bone—an increase in osteoclastic activity and a decreased bone formation by promoting osteoblast apoptosis. Another factor is elevation of the tumor necrosis factor (TNF) α which increases osteoclast-mediated bone resorption without concomitant increases in bone formation.

Once ART has been initiated, there is a consistent reduction in bone density especially in the hips, with an up to 6% reduction seen. Tenofovir fumarate based treatment has a much lower BMD effect compared to other regimens containing lamivudine and emtricitabine. Tenofovir decreases BMD through a persistent urinary loss of phosphates. In a meta-analysis tenofovir alafenamide had a similar tolerability, safety, and effectiveness to tenofovir fumarate and probably had less adverse events related to renal and bone density outcomes in the treatment of naive or experienced patients with HIV-1. Protease inhibitors, on the other hand, have also been associated with skeletal deterioration in most studies.

DIAGNOSIS OF BONE INVOLVEMENT

Modern technology has created many methods for evaluation of bone mineral density and quality. These include ultrasonography, CT scan, MRI scan and the Dual Energy X-ray Absorptiometry (DEXA) scan.

The DEXA is the most widely using densitometry technique, and is regarded to be the gold standard for measure into bone mineral density and diagnosing osteoporosis (Fig. 20.1). The scan requires only a few minutes of lying down on a table. DEXA of two sites is usually indicated, the spine and hip. The lateral spine and ward's triangle region of the hip should not be used for diagnosis, because these sites overestimate osteoporosis and results can be falsely positive.

The BMD values (in g/cm^2) are not used for diagnosing osteoporosis. Instead, a working group of the WHO proposed to define osteoporosis on the basis of the T-score. The WHO diagnostic criteria define osteoporosis in terms of a T-score below –2.5 and osteopenia when the T-score is between –2.5 and –1 (Table 20.1). In addition to the T-scores, DEXA reports also provide Z-scores, which are calculated similarly to the T-score, except that

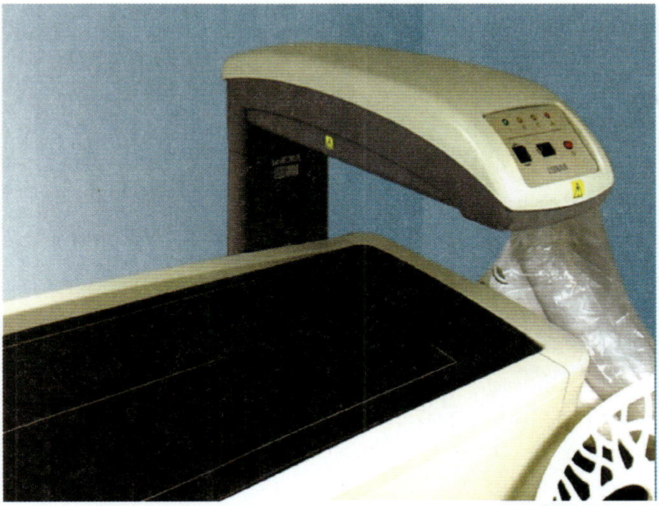

Fig. 20.1: DEXA machine.

Table 20.1: WHO classification of BMD according to the T-score.	
Name	***BMD (T-score)***
Normal	>–1
Osteopenia	–1 to – 2.5
Osteoporosis	At or below –2.5
Severe osteoporosis	Below –2.5 plus fragility fractures

the patient's BMD is compared with an age-matched (and race- and gender-matched) mean, and the result expressed as an SD score (Fig. 20.2). DEXA should not be repeated soon after the therapy as improvement may be seen only after 1–2 years.

FRAX Tool

The FRAX tool measures the probability of a major fracture for 10 years. The risk of fracture is calculated in men or women from various factors such as,

- Age
- Body mass index (BMI)
- A prior fragility fracture
- Parental history of hip fracture
- Current tobacco smoking
- Ever long-term use of oral glucocorticoids
- Rheumatoid arthritis
- Other causes of secondary osteoporosis
- Daily alcohol consumption of 3 or more units daily.

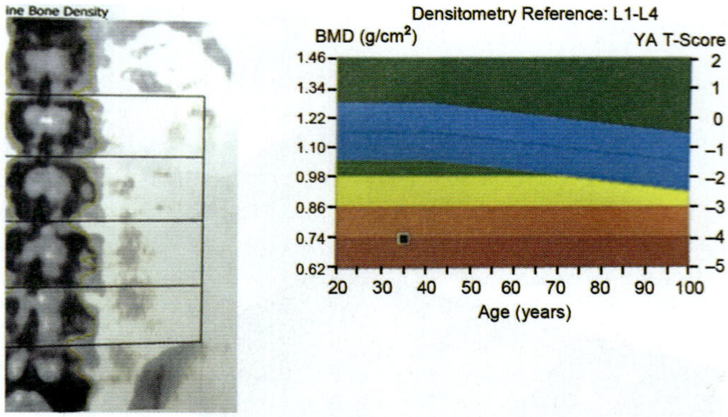

Fig. 20.2: DEXA report.

TREATMENT

Many antiresorptive agents including bisphosphonates, calcitonin, synthetic estrogen receptor modulators (SERMs), and denosumab (a monoclonal antibody against RANKL) are currently available for the management of osteoporosis. There is only one anabolic agent, teriparatide, available which promotes bone formation.

Oral bisphosphonate (alendronate, risodronate) is used in osteoporotic HIV infected individuals. However, their use may be limited by gastrointestinal side-effects such as esophagitis and their contribution to an already high pill burden due to highly active anti-retro viral therapy (HAART) and other prophylactic medications for treatment of opportunistic infections. As an alternative, annual zoledronic acid infusion has been shown to be well tolerated and to significantly increase BMD in HIV-infected individuals with osteoporosis.

CONCLUSION

- The results of various studies indicate a risk of low bone mineral disease in people living with HIV/AIDS.
- Despite national guidelines suggesting testing for bone health in PLHA, there are no large Indian data available for the above.
- Patients with HIV/AIDS are at risk of developing osteopenia/osteoporosis and should be classified as a high risk group for bone health.
- Tenofovir based ART isassociated with greater bone loss over the first few years compared with TDF-sparing regimens.
- Vitamin-D and calcium supplements should be incorporated as a part of treatment in PLHA patients.

SUGGESTED READING

1. Havens PL, Stephensen CB, Van Loan MD, et al. Vitamin D3 supplementation increases spine bone mineral density in adolescents and young adults with human immunodeficiency virus infection being treated with tenofovir disoproxil fumarate: a randomized, placebo-controlled trial. Clin Infect Dis. 2017 Aug 21.
2. Havens PL, Stephensen CB, Van Loan MD, et al. Decline in bone mass with tenofovir disoproxil fumarate/emtricitabine is associated with hormonal changes in the absence of renal impairment when used by HIV-uninfected adolescent boys and young men for HIV preexposure prophylaxis. Clin Infect Dis. 2017;64(3):317-25.
3. Lima AL, de Oliveira PR, Plapler PG, et al. Osteopenia and osteoporosis in people living with HIV: multiprofessional approach. HIV/AIDS (Auck). 2011;3:117-24.
4. Mastaglia S, Watson D, Bello N, et al. Vitamin D levels and their impact on mineral metabolism in HIV infected patients: an exploratory study. Clin Cases Miner Bone Metab. 2017;14(1):18-22.
5. Okonkwo RI, Weidmann AE, Effa EE. Renal and bone adverse effects of a tenofovir-based regimen in the treatment of HIV-infected children: a systematic review. Drug Safety. 2016;39(3):209-18.
6. Orkin C, Llibre JM, Gallien S, et al. Nucleoside reverse transcriptase inhibitor-reducing strategies in HIV treatment: assessing the evidence. HIV Medicine. 2018;19(1):18-32.
7. Panayiotopoulos A, Bhat N, Bhangoo A. Bone and vitamin D metabolism in HIV. Rev Endocr Metab Disord. 2013;14(2):119-25.
8. Weitzmann MN, Ofotokun I, Titanji K, et al. Bone loss among women living with HIV. Curr HIV/AIDS Rep. 2016;13(6):367-73.

CHAPTER 21

Coinfections with Hepatitis B and C

Ashish Kumar, Shrihari Anil Anikhindi

INTRODUCTION

Hepatitis B virus (HBV) infection is among the most common causes of chronic liver disease worldwide. India falls into the moderately high prevalence region with a carrier rate of around 3%. It is estimated to be especially higher in some tribal regions considered to be HBV hotspots. A study conducted in North India reported the prevalence of HBsAg to be 1% to 6% among blood donors and 2.6% to 9.5% in pregnant women.

With the arrival of the human immunodeficiency virus (HIV) epidemic, it is not uncommon to come across patients with HIV-HBV coinfection. Chronic Hepatitis B is seen in around 10% of the HIV infected patients. This is attributed to common modes of transmission of the two viruses. The highest rates of coinfection are reported from Asia and sub-Saharan Africa where the predominant mode of transmission is perinatal. In Western countries, coinfection is most commonly seen in high-risk groups like injection drug users and men having sex with men (MSM). Both HBV and HIV lead to chronic disease and the biggest challenge is that the presently available antiviral agents cannot eradicate both infections.

PATHOGENESIS

Hepatitis B virus is a non-cytopathic virus and hepatitis occurs due to the host immune response and not due to virus per se. Robust CD4+ and CD8+ responses are responsible for the clearance of infection in those who spontaneously recover from HBV infection. Whereas, a weak non-focused T cell response leads to establishment of chronic HBV infection.

Immunosuppression seen in HIV alters the natural history of HBV. The following features have been noted:

1. HBV DNA levels are higher in coinfected patients.
2. There is a strong risk of HBV reactivation in coinfected patients with the risk being associated with low CD4 cell counts.

3. Patients with documented resolution of HBV infection (loss of HBsAg) have been reported to have reappearance of HBsAg with HBV viremia in case of HIV coinfection.
4. Rates of spontaneous HBeAg clearance are lower in coinfections.

Clinical Syndromes

Acute HBV

Hepatitis B virus infections acquired during adulthood mostly resolve symptomatically after causing a brief flu like illness. Symptoms resolve in 90–95% of non-HIV infected patients within 4–6 weeks with formation of anti-Hepatitis B surface (HBs) antibody. These patients are considered immune. However in coinfected patients, anti-HBs antibody formation rate is much lower.

Chronic HBV

Failure of clearance of HBV by the body's defense mechanism leads to persistence of infection and subsequent incorporation of the viral genome into that of the host. Ongoing chronic inflammation leads to progressive liver injury eventually causing cirrhosis, hepatic decompensation and hepatocellular carcinoma. Chronic hepatitis B may show envelope (e) antigen positive or negative phases associated with relatively higher or lower viral loads respectively. Some patients show chronic carriage of HBs antigen without much inflammatory response. The HBs clearance rate in non-HIV infected carriers is around 2% per year. This rate is much lower in HIV infected patients.

Reactivation

Some patients with asymptomatic HBsAg carriage or even resolved HBV infection may present with reactivation of the virus. This scenario is especially common in HIV positive patients or those with other causes of immunosuppression. Sometimes reactivation may also occur due to immune reconstitution after initiating anti-retro viral (ARV) therapy.

Interpretation of the HBV Panel

The natural history of HBV infection is complex. Several antigen and antibody markers are present which in varying combinations are useful to determine the stage of the disease. Table 21.1 lists the panel of markers and their interpretation.

Treatment of HIV-HBV Coinfection

Very few studies have been conducted in HIV-HBV coinfected patients to formulate class I evidence. Most of the followed protocols are based on

Table 21.1: Interpretation of various HBV markers.

HBsAg	Anti-HBs	IgM anti-HBc	IgG anti-HBc	HBeAg	Anti-HBe	HBV DNA	Stage of infection
+	-	-	-	+	-	Low	Incubation
+	-	+	+	+	-	High	Acute HBV infection
+	-	+/-	+	+/-	-	High/Low	Chronic HBV infection
+	-	+/-	+	-	+	Low	Inactive carrier
-	+	+/-	+	-	+	Not detected	Resolved infection
-	+	-	-	-	-	Not detected	HBV vaccination

expert opinion. According to most recent guidelines, it is recommended to initiate treatment for both viruses in coinfected patients. This holds true for all patients with chronic hepatitis B, while in patients with acute hepatitis, therapy is indicated in patients who present with liver failure.

Acute HBV Infection

Most uncomplicated cases of acute HBV infection resolve spontaneously without any sequlae. Antiviral therapy in this setting has not shown to increase rates of HBsAg seroconversion, hence, any benefit is questionable. The only clinical setting in which anti-HBV therapy is indicated is in patients presenting with fulminant liver failure. Some studies have shown benefit of lamivudine therapy in this scenario. However, development of HIV resistance to lamivudine is a definite risk. Tenofovir and adefovir are associated with proximal renal tubular dysfunction. As around 20% of patients with acute liver failure will have some evidence of kidney injury; the use of tennfovir or adefovir for treating HBV is not indicated in these patients.

If a patient with fulminant liver failure is not already on ARV therapy, it is prudent to defer HIV treatment until stabilization of the liver status. In case the patient is already taking ARV therapy, lamivudine must be incorporated into the regimen and tenofovir/adefovir substituted.

Chronic HBV Infection

In coinfected patients with stable chronic hepatitis, therapy that is effective against both HBV and HIV is indicated. The use of an ARV regimen that includes two drugs also having activity against HBV is recommended. The preferred protocol is tenofovir plus either lamivudine or emtricitabine. It is important to avoid discontinuation of any drug unless significant adverse events/intolerance is noted. In case changing the ARV regimen is being considered, agents active against HBV must be the last to be stopped.

As in cases of HBV monotherapy, the aims of treatment for HBV in coinfection include:

- Clearance of HBsAg with anti-HBs seroconversion: this is the primary goal of treatment but rarely achieved. Hence, other secondary goals also need to be considered.
- HBeAg to anti-HBe seroconversion.
- Suppression to the lowest HBV levels.
- Reduction of liver inflammation.
- Prevention or delay of progression of fibrosis, cirrhosis and hepatocellular carcinoma.

Vaccination

Hepatitis B virus is a preventable disease as an excellent vaccine is available which provides high levels of protection. Anti-HBs titers of >10 IU/L are considered fairly protective while levels > 100 IU/L are considered completely protective against HBV infection. However in HIV infected patients, lower anti-HBs titers are achieved as compared to the normal population. It is recommended to obtain quantitative anti-HBs titers 1 to 2 months after the last vaccine series. Patients who have anti-HBs < 10 IU/L despite vaccination should be revaccinated.

Drug dosages

Drug	*Dose*	*Frequency*
Standard interferon	5 μ SC 10 μ SC	OD Thrice weekly
Pegylated interferon alfa-2a	180 μ SC	Once weekly
Lamivudine*	100 mg in HBV monoinfections 300 mg in HIV-HBV coinfections	OD OD
Adefovir	10 mg	OD
Telbivudine	600 mg	OD
Tenofovir/Disoproxil/ Fumarate*	300 mg	OD
Tenofovir/Alafenamide	25 mg	OD
Entecavir*	0.5 mg for nucleoside naïve patients 1 mg for decompensated cirrhotics 1 mg for patients previously treated with lamivudine	OD OD

* May need dose adjustment in CKD patients.

Lamivudine	
≥50	100 mg daily
30–49	100 mg first dose, then 50 mg daily
15–29	100 mg first dose, then 25 mg daily
5–14	35 mg first dose, then 15 mg daily
<5 or hemodialysis	35 mg first dose, then 10 mg daily
Adefovir	
≥50	10 mg daily
20–49	10 mg every other day
10–19	10 mg every third day
Hemodialysis patients	10 mg every week following dialysis
Telbivudine	
≥50	600 mg once daily
30-49	600 mg once every 48 hours
<30 (not requiring dialysis)	600 mg once every 72 hours
End-stage renal disease	600 mg once every 96 hours
Tenofovir	
≥50	300 mg every 24 hours
30–49	300 mg every 48 hours
10–29	300 mg every 72–96 hours
<10 with dialysis	300 mg once a week or after a total of approximately 12 hours of dialysis
<10 without dialysis	No recommendation
Entecavir	
Nucleoside naive	
≥50	0.5 mg daily
30–49	0.25 mg daily or 0.5 mg every 48 hours
10–29	0.15 mg daily or 0.5 mg every 72 hours
<10 or hemodialysis or continuous ambulatory peritoneal dialysis	0.05 mg daily or 0.5 mg every 7 days
Lamivudine refractory/resistant	
≥50	1 mg daily
30–49	0.5 mg daily or 1 mg every 48 hours
10–29	0.3 mg daily or 1 mg every 72 hours
<10 or hemodialysis or continuous ambulatory peritoneal dialysis	0.1 mg daily or 1 mg every 7 days

HIV-HCV COINFECTION

Disease Burden

The human immunodeficiency virus (HIV) and Hepatitis C virus (HCV) have emerged as important public health problems over the past few decades. Once unknown, they have of late attracted a large quantum of healthcare attention. According to the recent World Health Organization (WHO) estimates, 37 million people globally are infected with HIV, while the figure for chronic HCV infection is 115 million.

The HIV and HCV have similar modes of transmission, hence an overlap of affected populations is natural. More than 2 million people worldwide have HIV-HCV coinfection. HCV is the most common viral hepatitis seen in HIV infected patients. The most common cause of liver related mortality in HIV is chronic hepatitis.

The strongest risk factor associated with HIV-HCV coinfection is intravenous drug abuse. Other causes include patients requiring frequent blood transfusions like hemophiliacs, prison inmates and people with high risk behavior like men having sex with men (MSM). A Canadian health report published in 2001 showed the proportion of various risk factors for HIV-HCV coinfection (Fig. 21.1).

As compared to isolated infections, HIV-HCV coinfections pose a greater threat to the patient as they accentuate the pathology caused by each individual virus. Both viruses work in varying degrees of synchrony to produce greater damage to the host liver and immune systems.

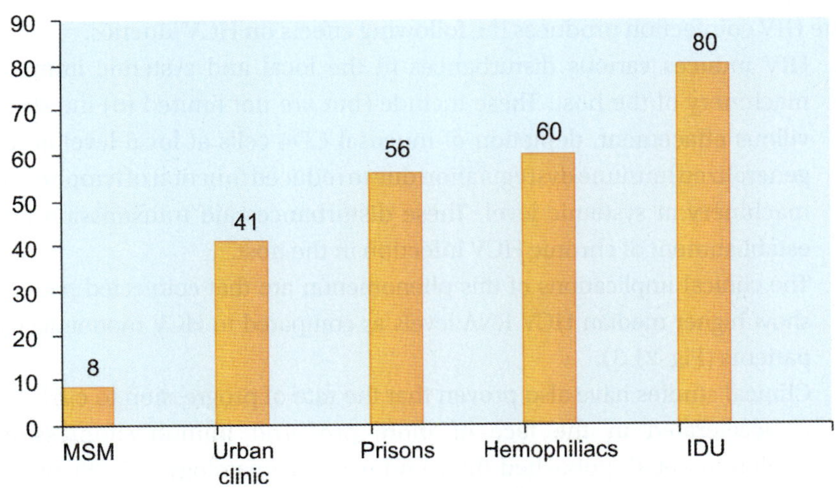

Fig. 21.1: Risk factors for HIV-HCV coinfection. (MSM: Men sex with men; IDU: Injection drug user).

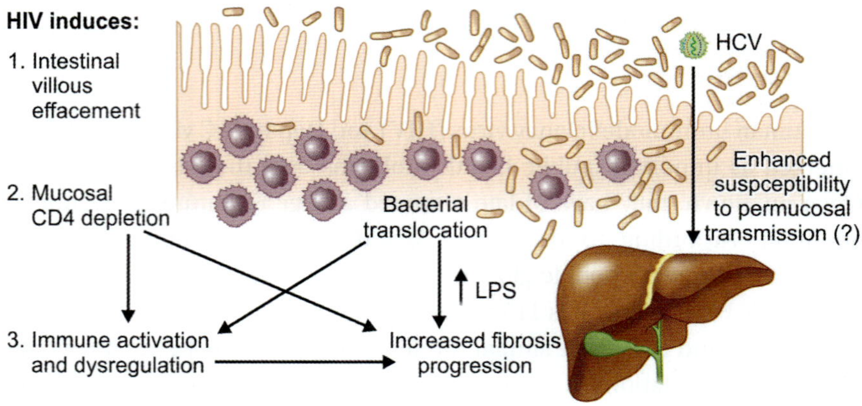

Fig. 21.2: Effect of HIV on HCV kinetics.

Effects of HCV on HIV Kinetics

The following effects on HIV kinetics are observed in cases of HCV coinfection:

1. HIV-infected patients with HCV coinfection have a faster progression to full blown acquired immune deficiency syndrome (AIDS).
2. Coinfected patients show slower CD4+ recovery than patients with HIV infection do alone.
3. Coinfected patients show slower immunological response to highly active anti-retro viral therapy (HAART) as compared to only HIV infected patients.

Effects of HIV on HCV Kinetics (Fig. 21.2)

The HIV coinfection produces the following effects on HCV kinetics:

1. HIV induces various disturbances in the local and systemic immune machinery of the host. These include (but are not limited to) intestinal villous effacement, depletion of mucosal CD4 cells at local level and a generalized immune dysregulation due to reduced function of lymphocyte machinery at systemic level. These disturbances aid transmission and establishment of chronic HCV infection in the host.
2. The clinical implications of this phenomenon are that coinfected patients show higher median HCV RNA levels as compared to HCV monoinfected patients (Fig. 21.3).
3. Clinical studies have also proven that the rate of progression to cirrhosis is accelerated in the face of more profound immunosuppression. Benhamou et al. published their findings in Hepatology in 1999, which clearly showed faster progression to cirrhosis in patients having lower CD4 cell levels and higher viral load (Fig. 21.4).

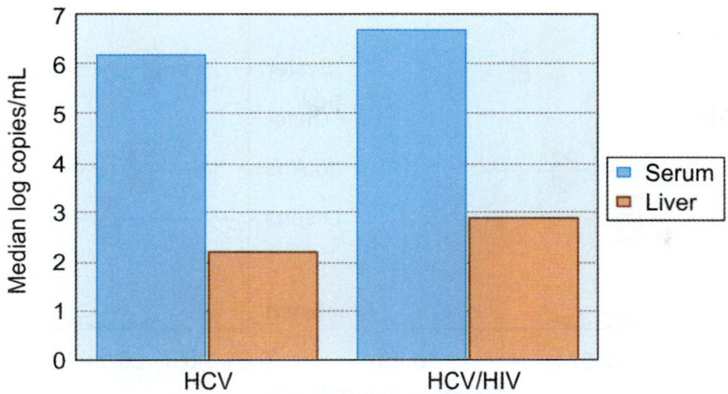

Fig. 21.3: Mean HCV RNA levels in HIV/HCV coinfection and monoinfected HCV patient.

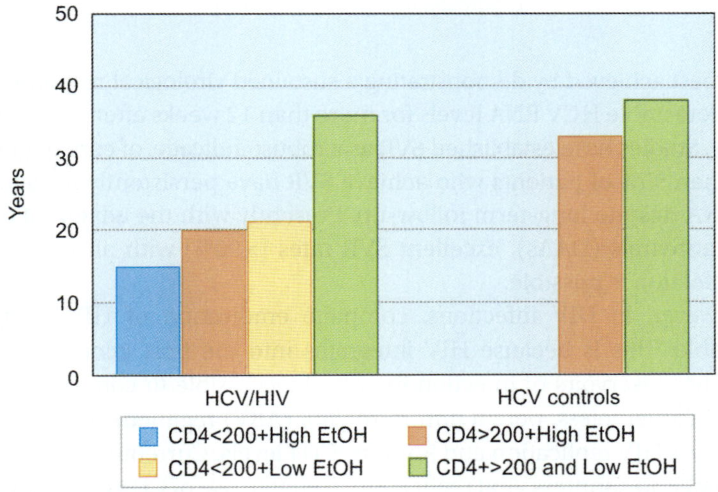

Fig. 21.4: Higher viral load and lower CD4 cell count are associated with acclerated progression to cirrhosis.

4. Meta-analyses have confirmed that progression to decompensated cirrhosis and end stage liver disease is much more common in coinfected patients (Fig. 21.5).
5. Other effects observed in coinfected patients include false negative antibody tests, lower rates of sustained virological response (SVR) for HCV treatment, increased psychiatric problems and higher incidence of insulin resistance/diabetes mellitus.

Treatment of HIV-HCV Coinfection

Principles of Treatment

Treatment goals in coinfected patients remain the same as with mono-infections. The goal of therapy in HCV is to achieve eradication of the virus.

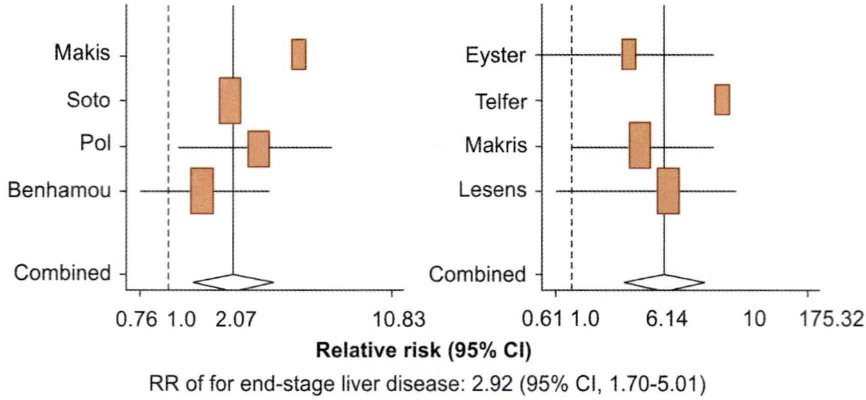

Fig. 21.5: Meta analysis data reveal that coinfection of HIV/HCV have higher progression to decompensation.

This is best achieved by demonstrating a sustained virological response (SVR), i.e. undetectable HCV RNA levels for more than 12 weeks after completion of therapy. Studies have established SVR as a robust indicator of cure of infection. More than 95% of patients who achieve SVR have persistently undetectable viral RNA despite long-term follow-up. Presently with the advent of directly acting antivirals (DAAs), excellent SVR rates (>90%) with all genotypes of HCV infection is possible.

However, in HIV infections, complete eradication of HIV is still not achievable. This is because HIV integrates into the host genome and also establishes reservoirs of infection in areas inaccessible to conventional drug therapy. Nonetheless, potent anti-retro viral (ARV) regimens have the ability to suppress HIV replication and improve CD4 levels. Currently the goal of HIV treatment is to suppress viral replication to enable rise of CD4 counts, which in turn translates to a lower incidence of opportunistic infections (Fig. 21.6).

Though the basic principles of treatment in coinfections remain the same, there are a few valid concerns in instituting treatment of coinfected patients. These include potential interactions among various drugs, increased drug toxicities and pill burden. While most guidelines recommend starting HCV therapy with similar principles and regimens as in HCV monoinfection, there has been some controversy regarding the timing of initiation of ARV therapy in coinfected patients.

Though there is strong evidence with randomized controlled trial backed data for initiation of ARV in all HIV-HCV coinfected patients irrespective of CD4 counts, some experts recommend following protocols:

- In ART-naive patients having CD4 counts >500 cells/mm^3, defer ARV therapy until completion of HCV treatment.
- In patients with CD4 counts <200 cells/mm^3, ARV therapy to be initiated promptly. In these patients, HCV therapy may be started after the patient is on stable ARV therapy.

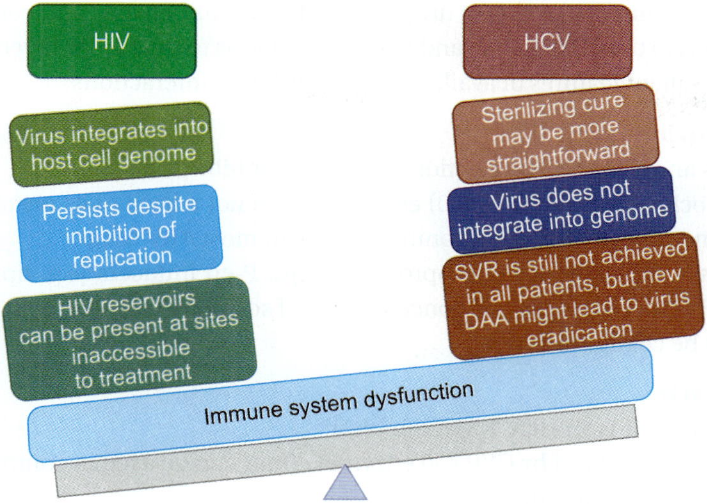

Fig. 21.6: HIV and HCV effect on immune system.

Treatment Regimens

Recommended ARV regimen in treatment naïve patients currently consists of:

1. Two nucleoside reverse transcriptase inhibitors (NRTIs) [Most commonly abacavir/lamivudine (ABC/3TC), tenofovir/alafenamide/emtricitabine (TAF/FTC), or tenofovir/disoproxil/fumarate/emtricitabine (TDF/FTC)]
2. In combination with third ARV drug from among the three drug classes
   a. Integrase strand transfer inhibitor (INSTI)
   b. Non-nucleoside reverse transcriptase inhibitor (NNRTI)
   c. Protease inhibitor (PI) including pharmacokinetic (PK) enhancer (booster) (cobicistat or ritonavir).

For HCV treatment; in the Interferon (IFN) era, treatment of HCV in HIV coinfected patients had very poor outcomes. As IFN is an immunomodulator, it depends on the host immune system to further its action. Thus, in immunosuppressed individuals with HIV infection, IFN treatment showed very poor SVR rates in the range of 20–40% for HCV therapy.

Introduction of directly acting antivirals (DAAs) over the last decade has completely transformed the landscape of HCV therapy. Excellent treatment outcomes are seen even in HIV coinfected patients. Currently the American Association for the Study of Liver Diseases (AASLD), the European Association for the Study of the Liver (EASL), and the Indian National Association for the Study of the Liver (INASL) recommend that patients with and without HIV coinfection be treated with the same HCV regimens. However, drug interactions need to be considered before starting any treatment for HIV and HCV concurrently. Initiation of HCV therapy along with ARV therapy requires a thorough understanding of drug-drug interactions between anti-retro viral therapies to treat HIV (ARV) and DAA medications to treat HCV. Given below are the salient features of available DAA's and their interactions

Sofosbuvir

- It is an HCV NS5B nucleotide polymerase inhibitor.
- Cytochrome P450 (CYP 450) enzyme system not related to its metabolism. Hence, it can be used in combination with most ARV drugs.
- It is a substrate of p-glycoprotein (P-gp). P-gp inducers [e.g. tipranavir (TPV)] decrease plasma concentration of sofosbuvir. Hence, both should not be coadministered.

Ledipasvir

- Ledipasvir is an HCV NS5A inhibitor
- Not metabolized by CYP 450 enzymes. Thus, can be used in combination with several ARV drugs.
- It is a P-gp substrate. Coadministering ledipasvir/sofosbuvir and ARV regimens containing tenofovir/disoproxil/fumarate (TDF) causes increased exposure to TDF. This is especially true when TDF is taken with a PI [boosted with either ritonavir (RTV) or cobicistat (COBI)]. If the drugs are coadministered, possibility of TDF-associated renal injury should be kept in mind.
- Inhibits breast cancer resistance protein (BCRP).

Daclatasvir

- Daclatasvir is an HCV NS5A inhibitor.
- It is a substrate of CYP3A. Strong inducers of CYP3A (e.g. efavirenz and nevirapine) decrease plasma levels of daclatasvir, thus reducing the drug's therapeutic effect. If coadministration is considered, dosage of daclatasvir should be increased to 90 mg OD.
- Plasma levels of daclatasvir may increase if coadministered with strong CYP3A inhibitors. If this regimen is considered then, dosage of daclatasvir should be reduced to 30 mg OD.
- It is an inhibitor of P-gp.
- It is an inhibitor of OATP1B1.
- It is an inhibitor of Breast Cancer Receptor Protein (BCRP).

Elbasvir/Grazoprevir

- Elbasvir is a NS5A inhibitor and grazoprevir is a protease inhibitor.
- Both elbasvir and grazoprevir are substrates of CYP3A. Coadministration with strong CYP3A inducers (e.g. EFV) may cause decreased plasma concentrations of elbasvir and grazoprevir. Hence, this combination is contraindicated.
- Coadministration of elbasvir and grazoprevir with strong CYP3A4 inhibitors may cause increased concentrations of elbasvir and grazoprevir and hence this combination is contraindicated.

- Both elbasvir and grazoprevir are substrates of P-gp.
- Both elbasvir and grazoprevir are of inhibitors of BCRP.
- Grazoprevir is also a substrate of OATP1B1/3 transporters.

PROD regimen

- Ombitasvir (NS5A inhibitor), paritaprevir (PI), ritonavir (pharmacokinetic enhancer), dasabuvir (NS5B inhibitor)
- Paritaprevir
  - It is a substrate and inhibitor of the CYP3A4.
  - It is a substrate and inhibitor of OATP1B1/3.
  - It is an inhibitor of UGT1A1.
  - It is a substrate of P-gp.
  - It is a substrate of BCRP.
- Ombitasvir
  - It is an inhibitor of UGT1A1.
  - It is a substrate of P-gp.
  - It is a substrate of BCR.
- Dasabuvir
  - It is a substrate of CYP2C8.
  - It is an inhibitor of UGT1A1.
  - It is a substrate of P-gp.
  - It is a substrate of BCRP.

Simeprevir

- Simeprevir is a NS3/4A protease inhibitor.
- It is a substrate and inhibitor of CYP3A4.
- It is a substrate and inhibitor of P-gp.
- It is an inhibitor of drug transporter OATP1B1/3.

The various drug-drug interactions for HIV/HCV therapy are shown in Tables 21.2 to 21.4.

Table 21.2: HCV DAAs and ARV NRTI interactions.

	Sofosbuvir	*Dac-latasvir*	*Ledipasvir*	*Elbasvir/ Grazoprevir*	*PROD*	*Sime-previr*
Lamivudine (3TC)	✓	✓	✓	✓	✓	✓
Abacavir (ABC)	✓	✓	✓	✓	✓	✓
Emtricitabine (FTC)	✓	✓	✓	✓	✓	✓
Tenofovir Disoproxil Fumarate (TDF)	✓	✓	✓	✓	✓	✓
Tenofovir Alafenamide (TAF)	✓	✓	✓	✓	✓	✓

Table 21.3: HCV DAAs and ARV PI interactions.

<table>
<tr><th></th><th>Sofosbuvir</th><th>Daclatasvir</th><th>Ledipasvir</th><th>Elbasvir/ Grazoprevir</th><th>PROD</th><th>Simeprevir</th></tr>
<tr><td>Atazanavir unboosted (ATV)</td><td>✓</td><td>✓</td><td rowspan="4">If PI used with TDF (NRTI) then monitor for TDF toxicity</td><td>✗</td><td>✗</td><td>✗</td></tr>
<tr><td>ATV/r or ATV/c Ritonavir or Cobicistat boosted</td><td>✓</td><td>↓ DCV dose to 30 mg/ day</td><td>✗</td><td>✗</td><td>✗</td></tr>
<tr><td>Darunavir boosted DRV/r or DRV/c</td><td>✓</td><td>✓</td><td>✗</td><td>✗</td><td>✗</td></tr>
<tr><td>Fosamprenavir boosted FPV/r</td><td>✓</td><td>✓</td><td>✗</td><td>✗</td><td>✗</td></tr>
<tr><td>Saquinavir boosted SQV/r</td><td></td><td>↓ DCV dose to 30 mg/ day</td><td></td><td>✗</td><td>✗</td><td>✗</td></tr>
<tr><td>Tiprenavir TPV/r</td><td>✗</td><td>?</td><td></td><td>✗</td><td>✗</td><td>✗</td></tr>
</table>

Table 21.4: HCV DAAs and ARV NNRTI interactions.

<table>
<tr><th></th><th>Sofosbuvir</th><th>Daclatasvir</th><th>Ledipasvir</th><th>Elbasvir/ Grazoprevir</th><th>PROD</th><th>Simeprevir</th></tr>
<tr><td>Efavirenz (EFV)</td><td>✓</td><td>↑ DCV dose to 90 mg/ day</td><td rowspan="5">If PI used with TDF (NRTI) then monitor for TDF toxicity</td><td>✗</td><td>✗</td><td>✗</td></tr>
<tr><td>Etravirine (ETR)</td><td>✓</td><td>↑ DCV dose to 90 mg/ day</td><td>✗</td><td>✗</td><td>✗</td></tr>
<tr><td>Nevirapine (NVP)</td><td>✓</td><td>↑ DCV dose to 90 mg/ day</td><td>✗</td><td>✗</td><td>✗</td></tr>
<tr><td>Rilpivirine (RPV)</td><td>✓</td><td>✓</td><td>✓</td><td>✗</td><td>✓</td></tr>
<tr><td>Dolutegravir (DTG)</td><td>✓</td><td>✓</td><td>✓</td><td>✓</td><td>✓</td></tr>
<tr><td>Raltegravir (RAL)</td><td>✓</td><td>✓</td><td></td><td>✓</td><td>✓</td><td>✓</td></tr>
</table>

Liver Transplantation in HIV-HCV Coinfected Patients

With the advent of highly efficacious ARV, HIV infected patients can now expect near normal life expectancies. As a result, the presence of HIV infection alone is not considered a contraindication for liver transplantation any more. Liver transplantation is indicated in decompensated cirrhotics and refractory complications arising due to liver cirrhosis like the hepatopulmonary syndrome, portopulmonary hypertension, etc. Certain HIV specific criteria for consideration of liver transplantation include:

- Absence of untreatable diseases
  - Progressive multifocal leukoencephalopathy
  - Chronic intestinal cryptosporidiosis
  - Multidrug-resistant systemic fungal infections
  - Primary CNS lymphoma
- Pretransplant HIV RNA suppressed on HAART to <50 copies/mL or predicted absence of HIV viremia on combined anti-retro viral therapy.
- CD4+ T cell count >100/mL.
- Absence of AIDS-defining illness.

Drug	*Dose*	*Frequency*
Sofosbuvir	400 mg *No dosage recommendation in CKD patients with eGFR< 30 mL/min/1.73 m^2	OD
Ribavirin	1000 mg for < 75 kg 1200 mg for > 75 kg	Two/three divided doses
Ledipasvir	90 mg	OD
Daclatasvir	60 mg 30 mg if coadministered with strong CYP3A inhibitors 90 mg if coadministered with moderate CYP3A inducers	OD OD OD
Elbasvir	50 mg	OD
Grazoprevir	100 mg	OD
Paritaprevir	75 mg	OD
Ombitasvir	12.5 mg	OD
Ritonavir	50 mg	OD
Dasabuvir	250 mg	OD
Simeprevir	150 mg	OD

In conclusion, HIV-HCV coinfection is a common entity owing to their shared mechanisms of transmission. Its incidence is increasing due to lifestyle changes and increased awareness. Coinfected patients have a more severe disease course with rapid progression to end stage liver disease.

Excellent treatment outcomes are now available with introduction of DAAs. Clinicians should be aware of the potential drug-drug interactions to choose appropriate therapy.

CONCLUSION

- Coinfections with HBV and HCV in HIV-infected patients are fairly common due to shared modes of transmission.
- There is synergism among these viruses; as a result infections usually tend to be more severe and protracted in coinfected patients as compared to those who are monoinfected.
- Treatment of HIV-HBV coinfection must involve an ARV regimen which includes at least 2 drugs active against HBV.
- Treatment of HIV-HCV confection involves use of similar principles for treating HCV monotherapy; except that drug-drug interactions have to be kept in mind and dosages modified accordingly.

SUGGESTED READING

1. Kim AY, Chung RT. Coinfection with HIV-1 and HCV—a one-two punch. Gastroenterology. 2009;137:795.
2. McGovern BH. Hepatitis C in the HIV-infected patient. J Acquir Immune Defic Syndr. 2007; 45(Suppl 2):S47.
3. Panel on Opportunistic Infections in HIV-Infected Adults and Adolescents. Guidelines for the prevention and treatment of opportunistic infections in HIV-infected adults and adolescents: Recommendations from the Centers for Disease Control and Prevention, the National Institutes of Health, and the HIV Medicine Association of the Infectious Diseases Society of America. http://aidsinfo.nih.gov/contentfiles/lvguidelines/adult_oi.pdf
4. Soriano V, Poveda E, Vispo E, et al. Hepatitis B in HIV-infected patients. Clin Liver Dis. 2013;17:489.
5. Thio CL. Hepatitis B and human immunodeficiency virus coinfection. Hepatology. 2009;49:S138.
6. Thomas DL, Shih JW, Alter HJ, et al. Effect of human immunodeficiency virus on hepatitis C virus infection among injecting drug users. J Infect Dis. 1996;174:690.

SECTION 7

Precautions

CHAPTER 22

Pre-exposure Prophylaxis

Kishan Majithiya, Atul Kakar

INTRODUCTION AND DEVELOPMENT

Approximately 36.7 million people across the world are suffering from human immunodeficiency virus (HIV)/acquired immunodeficiency syndrome (AIDS) including 1.8 million children below the age of 15 years. HIV infection may not be curable but it is preventable. In children, HIV infection usually occurs from their mothers during pregnancy or during breastfeeding. In adults, transmission is mainly through sexual intercourse [males with males (MSM), males with females] or via intravenous (IV) drug use by sharing needles with someone who is HIV positive.

To prevent the spread of HIV epidemic, several measures, like post-exposure prophylaxis and prevention of mother-to-child transmission (PMTCT), were introduced. However, despite these measures, the incidence of new infections increased rapidly throughout the world. This warranted the introduction of pre-exposure preventive measures.

PRE-EXPOSURE PROPHYLAXIS

This aims to prevent HIV infection by using oral anti-retro viral therapy given to people who are not previously infected.

INITIATION OF PRE-EXPOSURE PROPHYLAXIS

Post-exposure prophylaxis for prevention for HIV was already known. However, initially there were no studies with high quality of evidence for pre-exposure prophylaxis.

After the introduction of Tenofovir and Emtricitabine (FTC) as anti-retro viral agents, several studies were conducted to demonstrate their efficacy and side effects as pre-exposure prophylactic agents. These trials were conducted in high-risk population groups like homosexual men, heterosexual men and women, injection sharers and IV drug abusers.

The results of these trials showed that pre-exposure therapy was effective in reducing HIV transmission in HIV-negative persons who were at high risk of exposure, if taken on a regular basis and had minimal side effects.

Based on these results, the Centers for Disease Control and Prevention established guidelines for pre-exposure prophylaxis which were also adapted by the World Health Organization (WHO). Very recently WHO has also recommended the use of pre-exposure prophylaxis in pregnant and breastfeeding women who have a high risk of acquiring and transmitting infection.

INDICATIONS

Eligibility for pre-exposure prophylaxis includes those who are HIV-negative but have a high chance of acquiring infection, like

- Person with a ongoing sexual relationship with an HIV-infected partner.
- An HIV-negative male not in a monogamous relationship, who is not using barrier methods for sexual intercourse and who has a recent history of sexually transmitted infections (STIs) within last 6 months.
- Heterosexual man (behaviorally bisexual) who has unprotected sexual intercourse with multiple partners with unknown HIV status.
- Any person who has a history of drug and needle sharing within the last 6 months.
- HIV-negative pregnant women who are at substantial of HIV infection, as part of comprehensive PMTCT care.

EVALUATION OF PERSON BEFORE STARTING PRE-EXPOSURE PROPHYLAXIS THERAPY

- History and clinical examination
- History regarding previous exposure and STIs
- Hepatitis B virus and hepatitis C virus serology
- HIV testing
- HIV testing of the sexual partners of pregnant women before starting pre-exposure prophylaxis as PMTCT care
- Renal function tests including creatinine clearance.

GOALS OF PRE-EXPOSURE PROPHYLAXIS THERAPY

- To prescribe safe and effective prophylactic therapy to uninfected persons with high-risk behavior
- Educate patients about the therapy to maximize their safer use
- Education and support for therapeutic adherence
- Regular monitoring of patients to detect HIV infection, drug side effects, and also provide comprehensive behavioral therapy.

REGIMENS FOR PRE-EXPOSURE PROPHYLAXIS

There are two regimens:

1. Tenofovir disoproxil fumarate (TDF) 300 mg once a day
2. Tenofovir disoproxil fumarate 300 mg plus Emtricitabine (FTC) 200 mg once a day.

PRECAUTIONS WHILE PRESCRIBING PROPHYLAXIS THERAPY

- Do not substitute other anti-retro viral medications in place of TDF/FTC or TDF.
- Pre-exposure prophylaxis should always to be used as a daily regimen.

TIME TO ACHIEVE PROTECTION

After starting daily prophylaxis therapy, additional HIV prevention measures should be taken for seven days. Regular daily therapy provides high levels of protection. Time is needed to build-up protective levels of the drug in the blood and other tissues. Other methods to lower risk during this period include: adopting safer sexual practices, such as not having vaginal or anal intercourse, or using condoms for all vaginal and anal intercourse.

STOPPING OF PRE-EXPOSURE PROPHYLAXIS THERAPY

Pre-exposure prophylaxis therapy can be stopped 28 days after the last exposure to HIV and if they are no longer at substantial risk of acquiring HIV infection.

ADVERSE EFFECTS AND MANAGEMENT DURING THERAPY

Before starting the therapy, every patient should be explained about side effects of pre-exposure prophylaxis therapy. They should also be explained the features that indicate the possibility of acute kidney injury or acute HIV infection, which might need urgent evaluation. They should be thoroughly counseled regarding the need for monitoring the therapy and timely follow-up whenever indicated.

CLINICAL FOLLOW-UP AND MONITORING OF THERAPY

After starting pre-exposure prophylaxis therapy, patient follow-up is usually done once a month initially to assess early side effects of therapy and adherence.

Once the patient gets accustomed to the therapy, a 3-month follow-up should suffice. Monitoring should be as follows:

- HIV testing at least every 3 months to document HIV negativity of patient
- For assessment of side effects, treatment adherence, and risk behaviors
- Renal function tests and creatinine clearance monitoring at least every 6 months during therapy
- In the presence of pre-existing morbidity like hypertension or diabetes mellitus, renal function test (RFT) monitoring should be done more frequently
- Rise in serum creatinine is not the indication to withhold the therapy when clearance remains greater than or equal to 60 mL/minute
- If creatinine clearance shows a decreasing trend (but still ≥60 mL/min), nephrologist consultation and further evaluation should be done to find out the cause of the decreasing creatinine clearance
- Testing STI is recommended for adolescents and adults who are sexually active
- Once a year the patient should be assessed for the need to continue pre-exposure prophylaxis therapy.

CONCLUSION

- Pre-exposure prophylaxis therapy is highly effective measure with minimal side effects to prevent acquiring HIV infection in people with high exposure risk.
- Each and every patient with high exposure risk should be advised for prophylactic therapy after history, clinical examination and recommended investigations.

SUGGESTED READING

1. Grant RM, Anderson PL, McMahan V, et al. Uptake of pre-exposure prophylaxis, sexual practices, and HIV incidence in men and transgender women who have sex with men: a cohort study. The Lancet Infectious Diseases. 2014;14(9):820-9.
2. Grant RM, Lama JR, Anderson PL, et al. Preexposure chemoprophylaxis for HIV prevention in men who have sex with men. N Engl J Med. 2010;363:2587-99.
3. Molina JM, Capitant C, Spire B, et al. On-demand preexposure prophylaxis in men at high risk for HIV-1 infection. N Engl J Med. 2015;373(23):2237-46.
4. Seifert SM, Glidden DV, Meditz AL, et al. Dose response for starting and stopping HIV preexposure prophylaxis for men who have sex with men. Clin Infect Dis. 2015;60(5):804-10.
5. WHO implementation tools for pre-exposure prophylaxis 2017.

CHAPTER
23

Postexposure Prophylaxis

Sairam B, Atul Kakar

INTRODUCTION

Immediately after the discovery of human immunodeficiency virus (HIV) in the early 1980s, a major risk of transmission was identified among healthcare and sex workers. It was then that the universal precautions came into effect in the healthcare arena. Since its discovery, the disease incidence is on a rising trend worldwide, and other preventive measures such as vaccines have so far showed only mixed results and safe microbicides for blocking the virus per se are not yet available. However, HIV infection is not always an immediate consequence of exposure providing a window of opportunity for us to intervene and prevent the infection. A continuous research process has led to the formulation of *postexposure prophylaxis* (PEP) of HIV.

PROBLEM STATEMENT

The Centers for Disease Control and Prevention has stated that more than 380,000 needle-stick accidents happen every year throughout the world, in spite of all, the precautions that are being used. However, it has been estimated that the actual numbers may be even higher. Technical incompetence, a lack of proper understanding of risk factors, carelessness, work burden, and above all concern about the paperwork have led to a serious under-reporting of exposures among healthcare workers.

COURSE OF DEVELOPMENT

The first attempt at PEP started with Zidovudine (ZDV or AZT). All those who were exposed, irrespective of the amount of exposure, were treated with AZT with the hope of preventing infection. However, most of them succumbed to the adverse effect of the medication. With the invention of new drugs and continuous research, tenofovir and protease inhibitors started gaining popularity. They were found to be safer and better tolerated. But then due to a lack of guidance, healthcare workers and sex workers were forced to continue the same poorly tolerated, and guidelines recommended for the older agents. To address this issue, the New York Department of Health AIDS institute updated their older guidelines, so that newer anti-retro viral drugs could be promoted and brought into the picture for the safety and betterment of living standards. These guidelines have now been adopted worldwide and with the invention of newer drugs and formulations, this area is ready for further research work and development.

MANAGEMENT AND EVALUATION OF EXPOSURE

- The exposed body site should be cleaned immediately.
- Soap and water should be used to wash the wound.
- The wound should not be "milked".
- The mucous membrane should be flushed with water.
- Irritation of skin is to be avoided; hence, alcohol, hydrogen peroxide, or betadine should not be used.
- After contamination of the eye, immediate flushing with water is recommended.
- The oral cavity should be flushed several times, at least for 10–15 seconds each time, with an aqueous solution.
- After sexual exposure, soap and water should be used to wash the penis and the genital mucosa should be flushed with water after urination, to wash away any urethral contamination. Using enemas is not recommended.

Prompt initiation of PEP is recommended after any exposure to blood or any kind of potentially infectious material that can be from an HIV infected or from an HIV unknown source.

Occupational Exposure

The transmission of HIV through percutaneous inoculation, i.e. a break in the skin caused by a sharp object like a needle or glassware, occurs in approximately 0.3% of instances. The features of exposure that increase the rate of transmission include:

- A needle in contact with the source patient's blood vessel
- A deep needle stick
- An instrument with visible blood on its surface
- A source patient who has advanced HIV disease (Table 23.1).

Theoretically, any exposure that pierces the skin can transmit the infection, but the rate increases when the sharp object is contaminated with potentially infectious material and the clinician must be able to decide the significance of the exposure. Splashes of infectious material to the mucous membranes (e.g. conjunctivae or oral mucosa) or broken skin also may transmit HIV infection (estimated risk per exposure, 0.09%). Thus PEP is recommended in:

Table 23.1: Occupational exposure types and relative risks.

Exposure type	***Relative risk***
Deep needle stick	16:1
Fresh blood on penetrating instrument	5:1
Needle in contact with blood vessel	5:1
Advanced HIV in the source	6:1
Mucous membrane exposure	1:10
Exposure of damaged skin	1:10

- Splashes of blood or any potentially infected material or body fluid onto a mucosal surface.
- A break in the skin by a sharp object contaminated by blood or body fluid or any potentially infectious material.
- A nonintact skin exposed to body fluid or blood or potentially infectious material.
- Bite from a patient with visible bleeding from the mouth that also has caused bleeding in an exposed worker.

Nonoccupational Exposure

The risk of HIV transmission from nonoccupational exposure depends on the nature of exposure. The risks of sexual transmission are difficult to quantify. This is because these data are influenced by many factors and are mainly based on observational studies, like the presence or absence of concomitant genital ulcer disease, anal or cervical dysplasia, circumcision status, other sexually transmitted infections (STIs), viral load, and virulence. The estimated risk is 0.1–10% with anal intercourse while vaginal intercourse has a risk of 0.1–1%. Oral intercourse poses a comparatively smaller risk of HIV transmission, though proper reports are not yet available and there are case reports in the literature to prove it does pose some risk. The estimated risk of transmission associated with sharing needles, as in intravenous drug abusers, is approximately 0.67% per needle-sharing contact (Table 23.2).

Higher-risk Exposures

- Insertive and receptive anal or vaginal intercourse with a source known to be HIV-infected or whose HIV status is unknown.
- Sharing a needle with a source known to be HIV-infected or whose HIV status is unknown.
- Injuries with exposure to any potentially infected fluids from a source known to be HIV-infected or whose HIV status is unknown.

Table 23.2: Type of unprotected contact and its risk of transmission in non-occupational exposure.

Type of unprotected contact	*Risk of transmission*
Anal sex ▪ Receptive (source patient status—positive) ▪ Receptive (source patient status—unknown)	0.1–7.5% 0.06–0.49% 0.02–0.19%
Anal sex—insertive (source patient status—unknown)	0.05–0.15%
Vaginal sex—receptive	0.03–5.6%
Vaginal sex—insertive	Unknown probability
Oral sex	

Lower-risk Exposures

- Oral-vaginal contact (insertive and receptive)
- Receptive penile-oral contact with or without ejaculation
- Oral-anal contact (insertive and receptive)
- Insertive penile-oral contact with or without ejaculation
- Factors that increase risk:
  - High-viral load
  - Mucosal break
  - Bleeding and exposure to frank blood
  - Associated genital ulcer disease or other STIs.

Exposure—No Risk

- *Kissing*: Closed mouth kissing poses no risk while open mouth kissing has a minimal risk, which in turn depends on the presence of ulcers or mucosal bleeding.
- Mouth-to-mouth resuscitation, when there is no mucosal damage.
- Human bites without bleeding.
- Exposure to a sterile solid bore needle or lancet.
- Masturbation.

It is important to quote that compared to HIV, the rates of transmission for hepatitis C virus (HCV) are almost 10 times greater and are almost 100 times greater for hepatitis B virus (HBV).

TIMING AND DURATION OF POSTEXPOSURE PROPHYLAXIS

Ideally, PEP should be initiated within 2 hours of exposure. It should not be delayed for laboratory confirmation. The maximum duration within which PEP should be initiated for optimal efficacy has not yet been described. However, there is evidence in the form of animal studies to initiate PEP as soon after the exposure as possible for maximum efficacy. According to these studies, the effectiveness of PEP probably declines when initiated after 24–36 hours postexposure; however, there are no studies to confirm these findings in humans. Therefore, it is imperative that, if appropriate for the exposure, PEP should be started in spite of the interval exceeding 36 hours. With high-risk exposures, the literature suggests that PEP should be initiated even after 1 week, thus making use of even the slightest advantage, it has to provide under such circumstances. In such cases, administration of PEP should be individualized based on risk benefit analysis. Latest guidelines recommend PEP to be initiated only within 72 hours of exposure.

As far as the duration is concerned, studies have shown the efficiency of ZDV in animal and occupational exposures when administered for 4 weeks. Based on these study results, it is recommended that the PEP should be given for 4 weeks, if it is tolerated.

EFFICACY OF POSTEXPOSURE PROPHYLAXIS, BASED ON HUMAN AND ANIMAL TRIALS

No human study has been conducted to prove the efficacy of PEP. However, several studies have been done over the last decade, which have helped in defining the key aspects of PEP guidelines. The first which described the efficacy of PEP was a case control study, which showed a reduction in transmission of HIV after ZDV prophylaxis. Following this first study, several case reports and observational studies followed; however, a randomized case control study is not an option because of ethical issues. Along with all this evidence of successful elimination of transmission contrary findings, which have demonstrated the failure of PEP have also been published. Even after the introduction of the three-drug PEP, according to the 2005 guidelines, evidence of failure has been reported across the world, especially among men who have sex with men (MSM). Later studies included the use of anti-retro viral prophylaxis to prevent mother-to-child transmission. It was later realized that only those studies, which included on neonatal prophylaxis without treating the mother with anti-retro viral drugs could explain the success of PEP. Later animal studies were introduced to explain the efficacy of the PEP. These studies used the simian immunodeficiency virus (SIV) and updated the 2016 guidelines on PEP, to explain its potential benefits. Indirectly, these studies also had the advantage of examining various routes of administration of the same drugs and comparing their efficacy. They have also had the possibility of introducing newer anti-retro viral agents into prophylaxis giving an opportunity to improve the already existing guidelines. Recently, these studies have been proving the efficacy of the PEP in animals against the SIV. It has also been shown in a study that subcutaneous tenofovir after an intravenous (IV) loading dose, if administered within 24 hours, has a 100% potential in preventing infection. One of the studies has also shown a lower seroconversion rate after administration of tenofovir compared to other drugs. However, these results may not be seen in humans, as the strains and other conditions differ.

RISKS OF POSTEXPOSURE PROPHYLAXIS

The important concerns regarding PEP are:

- Otherwise healthy people are exposed to the short-term side effects of anti-retro viral drugs, if they are not HIV infected.
- Drug resistance, if seroconversion occurs in spite of PEP.
- People resort to usage of PEP and become wholly dependent on it instead of resorting to more effective, long-term behavioral changes.

RISK MODIFICATION AMONG USERS OF POSTEXPOSURE PROPHYLAXIS

There have been studies conducted across the world to look for any association of PEP with future risk factor modification. Some studies demonstrated a higher risk of condom less anal intercourse (CAI) and MSM after the introduction and use of PEP, while others have demonstrated no relationship between the two. However, no study has proved that the use of PEP has made a person change his risk modifiable behavior. This has called for the need for physicians duty to counsel patients for long-term prevention and not just administer PEP.

It has also been proved that behavior interventions when combined with PEP have shown a better compliance, completion rate, and also better reduction in indulgence in high risk behavior during and after PEP.

Recommended Nonoccupational/Occupational Postexposure Prophylaxis Regimen

Tenofovir 300 mg PO daily	+	Emtricitabine 200 mg PO daily
Raltegravir 400 mg PO twice daily	+	Dolutegravir 50 mg PO daily

- In renal insufficiency, the dosage of Tenofovir and Emtricitabine/ Lamivudine should be adjusted in patients with baseline creatinine clearance less than 50 mL/min.
- Fixed-dose combinations should not be used in exposed persons with renal failure, as they might need a dose adjustment.
- Tenofovir must be cautiously used in persons with renal insufficiency or in those taking nephrotoxic drugs.
- Lamivudine 300 mg PO daily may be substituted for emtricitabine. However, a fixed-dose combination is available when tenofovir is used with emtricitabine (Truvada 1 PO daily).

- Antacids are better avoided or used cautiously when Raltegravir is used.
- If the source is a known people living with HIV and AIDS (PLHA), past and current anti-retro viral therapy (ART) details, viral load, and resistance data (if available) may warrant the use of alternate regimen.

Advantages: Proven potency in HIV, efficacy similar to ZDV and protease inhibitors, fewer drug-drug interactions, favorable side effect profile, excellent tolerability, and ease of administration.

Tolerability is one of the most important advantages of the above regimen. It is for the above reason that a tenofovir-containing regimen is preferred over ZDV. The regimen also provides a theoretical advantage over protease inhibitors by acting even before the integration of virus with cellular DNA.

Preferred Alternative Nonoccupational/Occupational Postexposure Prophylaxis Regimen

Tenofovir 300 mg PO daily + Emtricitabine 200 mg PO daily

+

Darunavir 800 mg PO daily, or Atazanavir 300 mg PO daily, or Fosamprenavir 1,400 mg PO daily

+

Ritonavir 100 mg PO daily

Protease inhibitors have an extensive drug interaction because of cytochrome P450 interactions. For example, Atazanavir absorption is blocked by proton pump inhibitors. Clinicians, therefore, should assess these interactions before prescribing a protease inhibitor-containing regimen.

This regimen differs from the preferred regimen of Tenofovir + Emtricitabine/Lamivudine in the fact that it is less tolerable than the above one. However, its tolerability is significantly better than the ones containing ZDV.

Alternative Postexposure Prophylaxis Regimens Following Occupational and Nonoccupational Exposure

- Tenofovir + Emtricitabine + Zidovudine
- Tenofovir + Emtricitabine + Lopinavir/Ritonavir
- Zidovudine + Lamivudine + Protease inhibitors*

*One of the following Ritonavir-boosted—Darunavir, Atazanavir, Fosamprenavir, or Lopinavir.

Lopinavir/Ritonavir combination has a little benefit over Raltegravir or Dolutegravir. Studies have also proved other Ritonavir-enhanced protease inhibitors to be as efficient as the Lopinavir–ritonavir combination.

Guidelines recommend a three-drug regimen for PEP in view of its enhanced effectiveness. However, if tolerability is a concern, a two-line regimen is considered to be better than discontinuing the course. Studies have showed that ZDV monotherapy can inhibit 81% of seroconversion, thus reminding us of the fact that any active retroviral agent can bring about the necessary change in seroconversion.

HIV PREVENTION COUNSELING

Although PEP is efficacious, it is not 100% effective in preventing HIV. Healthcare providers should also take responsibility to address the needs of behavioral interventions in the patients during and after PEPs. They should also identify the ongoing risk behavior and help patients in preventing the exposure to infection. The assessment should include nonjudgmental, frank questions about illicit drug use, alcohol use, and sexual behavior.

The incidence of the disease in people with exposure is low, however, the mental stress that the exposed person experiences is substantial. Although a low risk exists for HIV transmission even if they are actually infected, the exposed person should be warned about the secondary transmission, which might further strain their already troubled minds. Therefore, it is the duty of the physician to address the stress factor that is created in the exposed person, which becomes an important element of PEP. They should be made aware of the first 6–12 weeks of exposure in which most infected person seroconvert, and should be encouraged to adopt certain measures to prevent secondary transmission. Sexual abstinence, postponement of pregnancy, use of condoms, refrainment from organ blood or semen donation should be advised. In breastfeeding women, discontinuation from the same is to be advised, as it not only serves as the means of transmitting infection, but also the drugs like nucleoside reverse transcriptase inhibitors (NRTIs) can be transmitted to the child, exposing them to toxicity.

Exposed individuals should be advised to seek medical help in case of any acute illness they experience during the PEP. Fever, myalgia, malaise, fatigue, rash, or lymphadenopathy may actually indicate acute HIV infection but may also be due to another medical conditions or drug reactions.

Before administration of PEPs, the exposed person should be aware of certain information:

- A combination drug regimen is recommended because of increased potency and concerns about drug-resistance.
- Knowledge about the efficacy of drugs used for PEP is limited.
- The short-term toxicity of anti-retro viral drugs is usually limited but serious adverse events have occurred in persons taking PEP.
- Data regarding toxicity of anti-retro viral drugs in persons without HIV infection or in pregnant women are limited.

Exposed individuals for whom PEP is not recommended should be informed that the potential side effects and toxicity of taking PEP outweigh the negligible risk of transmission posed by the type of exposure.

FOLLOW-UP AFTER OCCUPATIONAL EXPOSURE

Postexposure prophylaxis is to be taken for 4 weeks with regular monitoring of certain parameters. A clinical visit is recommended at least twice—(1) one for a baseline check and (2) the other at 4 weeks after starting treatment.

- HIV testing is recommended to be done at the baseline visit—week 4 and week 12.
- HBV and HCV testing should be done at the baseline visit.
- Pregnancy testing is recommended to be done during the baseline visit.
- CBC, RFT, LFT to be monitored at the baseline visit, week 2 and week 4.
- In case of sexual exposure, testing for other STIs is recommended at the baseline visit and at 4 weeks.

Pregnant Women

No study has yet come up with recommendations for ART in an HIV-negative woman. However, there are studies available to know the drugs contraindicated or to be cautiously used during pregnancy.

Efavirenz is a category D drug that is recommended to be avoided in first-trimester pregnancy and in women in the childbearing age group who might get pregnant during the course of PEP.

A stavudine-didanosine combination should be avoided, as it causes fetal malformations because of lactic acidosis.

Indinavir is associated with the risk of nephrolithiasis and so is contraindicated in pregnant women.

Based on clinical experience with ARTs, PEPs should ideally be started within 2 hours of exposure in pregnant women. They should be counseled regarding the risks and benefits involved, to herself and also to the fetus. It is important to mention that in addition to the risk of seroconversion, the high-viral load in acute retroviral syndrome also increases the risk of transmission to breastfeeding infant or the fetus.

Context of Pre-exposure Prophylaxis

Postexposure prophylaxis need not be given to person who is already on pre-exposure prophylaxis (PrEP) with a good compliance. However, if the compliance is poor and the patient has not taken his drug for 1 week, PEP is indicated.

Tables 23.3 and 23.4 summarize the occupational and nonoccupational exposure and requirement of PEP.

Occupational Exposure (Table 23.3)

Table 23.3: An overview on occupational exposure.

Recommended	*Not recommended*	*Considered*
Percutaneous needle–stick injuries	Percutaneous contact with body fluids other than blood	Superficial injury
Deep injury	Contact of intact skin with blood	
IV injections with shared needles	Contact of skin with body fluid other than blood	
High-viral load in source		

(IV: Intravenous).

Nonoccupational Injury (Table 23.4)

Table 23.4: An overview on nonoccupational injury.

Recommended	*Not recommended*	*Considered*
Transfusion of HIV-containing blood products	Kissing	Oral sex with ejaculation with an HIV-infected person
Unprotected receptive sex with an HIV-infected person	Other contacts without semen or blood mucus membrane contact	
Sharing contaminated needles	Accidental needle–stick injury	

CONCLUSION

- PEP guidelines are available to decrease the incidence of HIV infection through timely delivery of combination of drugs.
- CDC and WHO guidelines do not recommend PEP in persons with negligible exposure and those who seek care after 72 hours of exposure.
- Combination of drugs is recommended as preferred regimen over monotherapy.
- Proper counseling about the adverse effects helps to ameliorate the side effects and also improves the adherence.
- Additional medical and psychosocial support along with PEP can bring down the HIV incidence considerably.

SUGGESTED READING

1. Centre for Disease Control and Prevention. Updated Guidelines for Antiretroviral Postexposure Prophylaxis After Sexual, Injection Drug Use, or Other Nonoccupational Exposure to HIV—United States, 2016. https://www.cdc.gov/hiv/risk/pep/index.html.
2. New York State Department of Health AIDS Institute. HIV Prophylaxis Following Non-Occupational Exposure Including Sexual Assault New York, NY: New York State Department of Health AIDS Institute; 2014: available at http://www.hivguidelines.org/clinical-guidelines/post-exposure-prophylaxis/hiv-prophylaxis-following-nonoccupational-exposure/.
3. World Health Organization. Joint WHO/ILO guidelines on Post Exposure Prophylaxis to prevent HIV infection. https://www.who.int/hiv/pub/guidelines/psp/en.

SECTION 8

Miscellaneous

CHAPTER 24

Palliative Care in HIV

Veronique Dinand, Atul Kakar

INTRODUCTION

As retroviral drugs are being made available for human immunodeficiency virus (HIV) patients, more and more people living with HIV/AIDS are living longer. For many of these patients palliative care should be integrated with definitive care. Palliative care is an interdisciplinary approach, which improves quality-of-life of the patient and also caters to the need of his or her relatives.

COMPONENTS OF PALLIATIVE CARE

The various important components of palliative care are ethical, psychosocial, spiritual, and physical. The approach is integrated with ongoing treatment for HIV/AIDS (Figs. 24.1 and 24.2).

Its general principles:

- To relieve pain
- To provide symptomatic relief from distressing symptoms

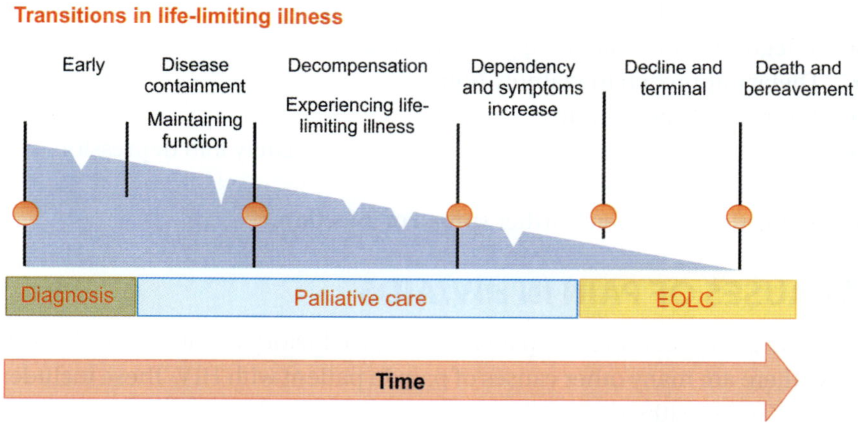

Fig. 24.1: Palliative care and end of life care (EOLC)—the continuum.

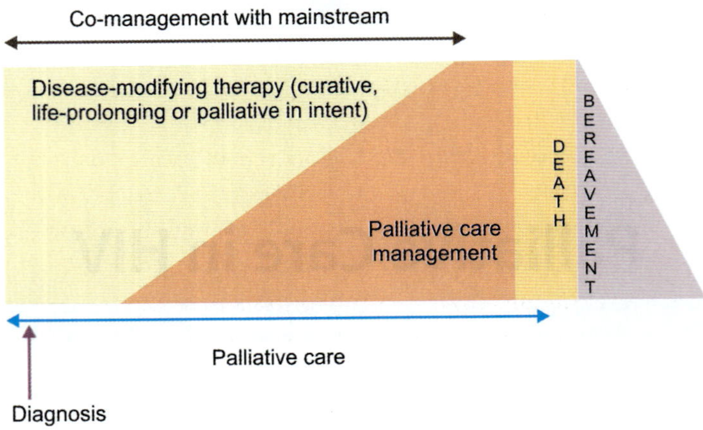

Fig. 24.2: Integrating palliative with curative care in HIV.

- It intends neither to hasten nor to postpone death
- Provide psychological support to the patient and his family
- To discuss and address any spiritual distress with the patient and his family
- To provide support to the patient and family in coping with the illness and treatment
- To improve the quality-of-life of the patient.

Whereas in the pre-anti-retro viral therapy (ART) era HIV/AIDS had a rapid fatality due to opportunistic infection the scenario has now changed. HIV/AIDS is now taken as a manageable chronic disease. Palliative care in HIV/AIDS addresses the following considerations:

- Comorbidities of hepatitis B and C
- Malignancies
- Symptoms, which have an effect on the quality-of-life
- Support to adhere to medication prescribed
- Integrating medical therapy with palliative care
- Dietary approach to malnutrition
- Forming support groups
- Treating mental and psychiatric aspects like anxiety and depression
- Support for legal services
- Education to prevent further spread of infection.

CAUSES OF PAIN IN HIV/AIDS

Chronic pain is common in patients who give history of substance abuse in HIV. There are many other causes of pain in patient with HIV. These include:

- HIV neuropathy
- HIV arthropathy

- ART induced neuropathy/pancreatitis
- Malignancy associated with neuropathy/myopathy
- Musculoskeletal pain due to HIV-wasting syndrome
- Wound pains due to secondary infection.

Human immunodeficiency virus infection itself can be associated with pain due to neurotoxicity. There are many barriers to treat pain in HIV. The most important is due to a lack of knowledge among physicians especially about opioid use. Many physicians are concerned about addiction, adjuvant therapy such as antidepressants, anticonvulsants, and muscle relaxants. The model of pain is shown in Figure 24.3. This pain ladder has been developed by the WHO. The basic step is to start with nonopioids for mild pain, weak opioids for moderate pain, and strong opioids for severe pain. Step 4 consists of interventional analgesics.

MULTIDISCIPLINARY APPROACH

Palliative care in HIV includes many specialists from medicine, nursing, psychology, social work, alternative medicine, and physical therapy. The team should be well-versed about distressing symptoms of HIV.

Patients with advanced HIV may complain of one or more of following symptoms:

- Anxiety, agitation, anorexia
- Bony pain, backache
- Chronic pain, cough
- Decubitus ulcer, delirium, dementia, diarrhea, dry mouth, dry skin, dyspnea
- Fever, fatigue

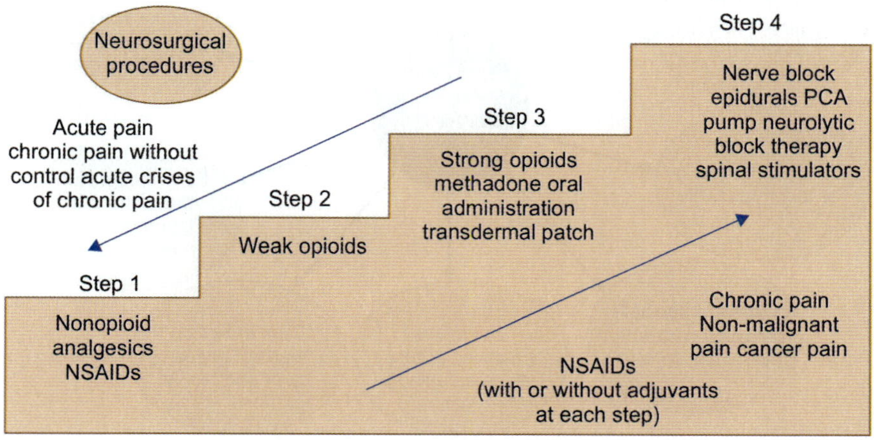

Fig. 24.3: The WHO pain ladder.

- Hiccups
- Weaknesses, weight loss
- Sleep disturbance, vomiting, pruritus.

COMMUNICATION SKILLS

The staff involved in palliative care should have good communication skills. They should clearly explain the treatment options and prognosis. The person involved in counseling should have the capacity to listen carefully and understand issues from the patient and his or her family members (Fig. 24.4).

END OF LIFE CARE

Even though mortality from HIV/AIDS has dramatically reduced with the advent of protease inhibitor therapy, patients ultimately die. In order to provide good end of life care, excellent symptom management is complemented by psychosocial and spiritual support to the patient and relatives. End-of-life care for persons with HIV/AIDS requires compassionate communication with the patient and relatives. Talking about death is difficult for the treating team and the patient and relatives. However, it is an important to discuss advanced care planning, tailored to individual needs and wishes. Writing a living will and giving advanced directives as to the preferred place

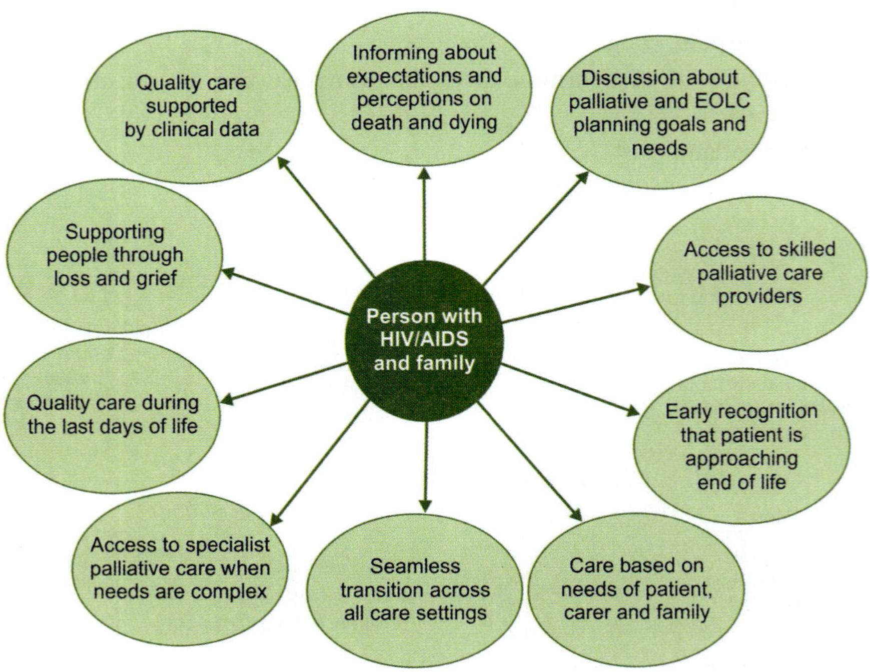

Fig. 24.4: End of care for HIV/AIDS patients and their family.

of care, non-resuscitation decisions, avoidance of futile treatment, etc. play an important role in the quality of death that will be achieved. But those directives do not replace the on-going communication between physicians and other team members, patients and relatives. Figure 24.4 gives end of life care for HIV patients.

Qualities of a Good Death

- Having control over the dying process
- Pain-free death
- Engagement with religion or spirituality
- Experiencing emotional well-being
- Having a sense of life-completion or legacy
- Having a choice in treatment preferences
- Experiencing dignity in the dying process
- Having family present and saying goodbye
- Quality of life during the dying process
- Good relationship with healthcare providers.

Bereavement Care

Bereavement care after the demise includes helping with formalities and providing bereavement counseling. The healthcare team ought to be empathetic and supportive of the family. Care and understanding at this time assists the family in coping with grief and makes them feel that they loved and cared for the patient in the best possible way.

CONCLUSION

Palliative care in HIV/AIDS should be an interdisciplinary effort, which aims to improve the quality-of-life of a person with AIDS.

It aims to provide psychosocial and spiritual support to the patient and relatives in a coordinated manner.

It is also important to remember that pain is under reported and under treated in many HIV patients.

SUGGESTED READING

1. Chu C, Selwyn PA. An epidemic in evolution: the need for new models of HIV care in the chronic disease era. J Urban Health. 2011;88(3):556-66.
2. Fausto JA, Selwyn PA. Palliative care in the management of advanced HIV/AIDS. Prim Care. 2011;38(2):311-26.
3. Huang YT. Challenges and responses in providing palliative care for people living with HIV/AIDS. Int Palliat Nurs. 2013;19(5):218.
4. Merlin JS, Bulls HW, Vucovich LA, et al. Pharmacologic and non-pharmacologic treatments for chronic pain in individuals with HIV: a systematic review. AIDS Care. 2016;28(12):1506-15.

CHAPTER 25

Immune Reconstitution Inflammatory Syndrome

Darshit Shah, Atul Kakar

INTRODUCTION

Immune reconstitution inflammatory syndrome (IRIS) is a term used to describe a set of inflammatory disorders, which is characterized by paradoxical worsening of previously existing infectious processes, treated or in a subclinical state by the initiation of highly active anti-retro viral therapy (HAART).

Immune reconstitution inflammatory syndrome can be:

- *Paradoxical IRIS* in which there is deterioration of a previously existing infection.
- *Unmasking IRIS* in which there is worsening of a previously unrecognized infection.

PATHOGENESIS

Human immunodeficiency virus (HIV) has a half-life of 1–4 days. Following initiation and continuation of HAART for 1–2 weeks, the HIV viral burden may show more than a 90% reduction of its previous value. Recession of the viral load is inversely related to the rise of immune effector cells. This reduction of viral load continues for the next 8–12 weeks following which it stabilizes.

The recovery of CD4 T lymphocytes following HAART is biphasic. The initial rise is due to an increase in the number of CD45RO memory cells and the secondary rise occurs following thymopoiesis. Following the initiation of HAART, there is expansion of the CD8 T lymphocytes, which later on stabilizes as the memory CD8 cells decline subsequently to be substituted by CD8 T lymphocytes.

Immune reconstitution inflammatory syndrome is usually seen in HIV-infected patients; however, it can also be seen in a small subset of HIV noninfected individuals under the following conditions:

- Corticosteroid withdrawal
- Cessation of anti-tumor necrosis factor (TNF)-alpha therapy
- Improvement of neutropenia following cytotoxic chemotherapy (Flowchart 25.1).

Flowchart 25.1: Classification of immune reconstitution inflammatory syndrome (IRIS).

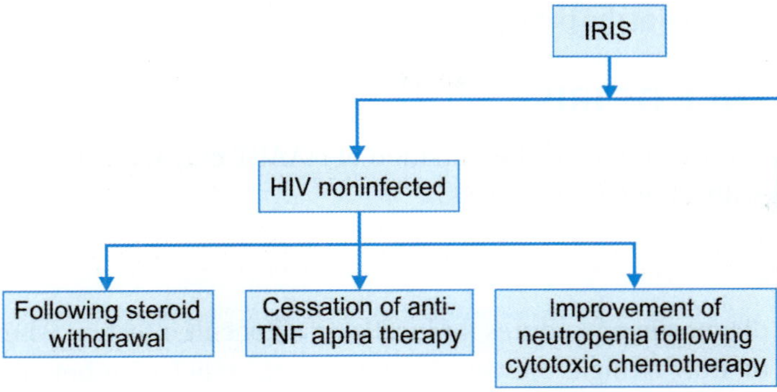

(TNF: Tumor necrosis factor).

The common organisms associated with IRIS are:

- *Mycobacterium tuberculosis*
- *Mycobacterium avium complex*
- *Cytomegalovirus*
- Herpes simplex virus
- Human herpes virus 8
- Hepatitis B virus
- *Cryptococcus*
- *Pneumocystis.*

RISK FACTORS

- Low baseline CD4 counts (<100 cells/μL)
- High-HIV ribonucleic acid (RNA viral load).

DIAGNOSIS

The following criteria are required for the diagnosis of IRIS:

- AIDS-positive patient with low-CD4 counts (often <100 cells/μL) except tuberculosis where IRIS can occur with CD4 counts more than 200 cells/μL.
- With the initiation of HAART, there should be a decline in viral load together with boosting of the immunological response.
- There should be a temporal association between the starting of HAART and onset of clinical features.
- There should not be any evidence of:
  - Drug allergy
  - Drug-resistant infection
  - Bacterial superinfection
  - Adverse drug reaction
  - Drug–drug interaction

- Malabsorption
- Noncompliance of the patient.

OCCURRENCE OF IRIS

The occurrence of IRIS following the initiation of HAART may range from 29 days to 99 days with a median of 48 days.

CAUTION

Avoid invasive diagnostic procedures for localizing an occult infection when the suspicion of IRIS is high. However, symptomatic relief of tubercular lymphadenitis is advocated by localized drainage with appropriate cultures.

DIFFERENTIAL DIAGNOSIS (FLOWCHART 25.2)

- Abacavir hypersensitivity is seen in patients of HLA-B*5701.

Flowchart 25.2: Differential diagnosis of immune reconstitution inflammatory syndrome (IRIS).

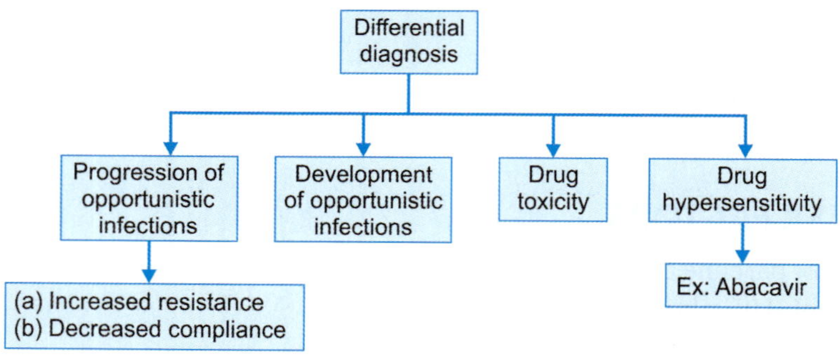

CLINICAL FEATURES

IRIS with Tuberculosis

Pulmonary Tuberculosis

- Fever
- Weight loss
- Malaise
- Respiratory distress.

Radiological Findings

- New parenchymal opacities
- Enlargement of intrathoracic lymph nodes.

Extraparenchymal Tuberculosis

- Worsening lymphadenopathy
- New pleural effusion
- Worsening of meningitis
- Tuberculoma expansion.

TREATMENT

- Nonsteroidal anti-inflammatory drugs (NSAIDs) can be given.
- In moderate-to-severe disease, corticosteroids can be used for 1–2 weeks with rapid tapering over 1–2 weeks.

IRIS in patients infected with *Mycobacterium tuberculosis* occurs usually within the first 2 months of the initiation of HAART.

HIV WITH NONTUBERCULOUS MYCOBACTERIA

Clinical Features

- Painful lymphadenopathy
- Fever.

Investigations

- Blood culture sterile
- Bone marrow culture sterile
- Lymph node biopsy reveals granulomatous infection.

When to Initiate Anti-retro Viral Therapy in Patients with Tuberculosis?

Anti-retro viral therapy (ART) should be initiated after 2 weeks of initiation of antituberculosis treatment (ATT) to reduce the risk of development of IRIS.

What to Do if IRIS Occurs (Flowchart 25.3)?

When anti-retro viral therapy is initiated in HIV patients, there are immunopathological changes which occurs, these are also called paradoxically reaction. Tuberculosis IRIS is a common setting which should be known to the clinicians. Two important risk factors are lower absolute CD4 cell counts and shorter interval between starting of ART and antitubercular treatment.

When IRIS is mild, nonsteroidal anti-inflammatory drugs should be used. It can reduce inflammation and fever in this condition. Surgical procedures like aspiration or incision of the tender lymph nodes may be done. Inhalation of steroids helps in presence of bronchospasm.

Flowchart 25.3: Management of immune reconstitution inflammatory syndrome (IRIS).

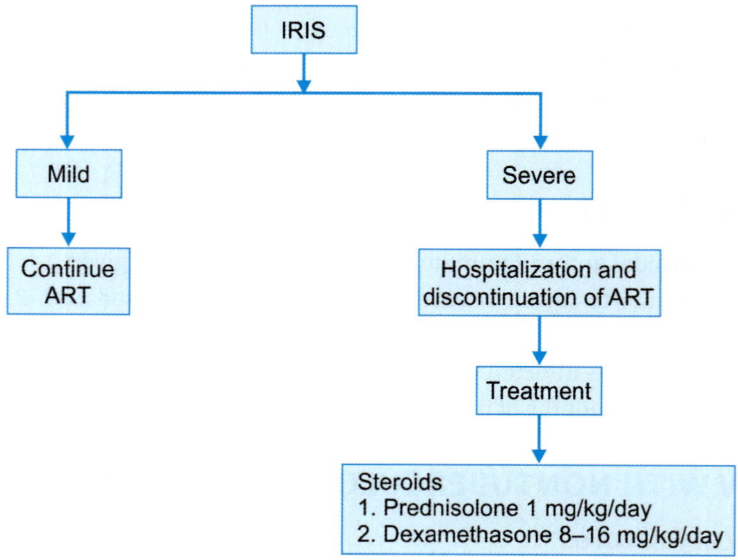

(ART: Anti-retro viral therapy).

Corticosteroids have been used for many years in special setting in tuberculosis. The drug has shown to reduce incidence of death especially in severe cases of tubercular meningitis. In some studies, they have been used in management of tubercular pericarditis to prevent constructive pericarditis. In case IRIS is severe and associated with Mycobacterium, prednisolone at a dose of 1-2 mg/kg or equivalent for 1-2 weeks can be beneficial. The physicians should avoid its use in cryptococcal meningitis and kaposis sarcoma associated IRIS. Close monitoring should be kept on blood sugars, blood pressure, avascular necrosis, worsting of infection or new onset of infection. Severe IRIS should be managed by HIV caregiver. Cryptococcal meningitis associated raised intracranial pressure can be managed by therapeutic lumbar puncture.

PREVENTION

- Identify opportunistic infections and treat them 1-2 months before initiation of ART.
- If the patient has *M. tuberculosis* infection with CD4 counts less than 100 initiate ART after 2 weeks.
- If the patient is having *M. tuberculosis* infection andthe CD4 counts are more than 100 initiate ART after 2 months.

CONCLUSION

- IRIS is a term, which is characterized by paradoxical worsening of previously existing infectious processes by the initiation of HAART.
- IRIS is usually seen in HIV-infected patients; however, it can also be seen in a small subset of HIV noninfected individuals following corticosteroid withdrawal, cessation of anti-TNF alpha therapy and improvement of neutropenia following cytotoxic chemotherapy.
- *Mycobacterium tuberculosis* and nontubercular mycobacteria are commonly associated with IRIS; however, IRIS can occur with other organisms as well.
- Risk factors include low baseline CD4 counts (<100 cells/μL) together with a high-HIV RNA viral load.
- Occurrence of IRIS following initiation of HAART may range from 29 days to 99 days with a median of 48 days.
- ART should be initiated after 2 weeks of the initiation of ATT to reduce the risk of the development of IRIS.
- Treatment includes NSAIDs for mild disease and corticosteroids for moderate-to-severe disease.

SUGGESTED READING

1. Antonelli LR, Mahnke Y, Hodge JN, et al. Elevated frequencies of highly activated CD4+ T cells in HIV+ patients developing immune reconstitution inflammatory syndrome. Blood. 2010;116:3818.
2. Breton G, Duval X, Estellat C, et al. Determinants of immune reconstitution inflammatory syndrome in HIV type 1-infected patients with tuberculosis after initiation of antiretroviral therapy. Clin Infect Dis. 2004;39:1709.
3. Cooney EL. Clinical indicators of immune restoration following highly active antiretroviral therapy. Clin Infect Dis. 2002;34:224.
4. Grant PM, Komarow L, Andersen J, et al. Risk factor analyses for immune reconstitution inflammatory syndrome in a randomized study of early vs. deferred ART during an opportunistic infection. PLoS One. 2010;5:e11416.
5. Günthard HF, Saag MS, Benson CA, et al. Antiretroviral drugs for treatment and prevention of HIV infection in adults: 2016 recommendations of the International Antiviral Society-USA Panel. JAMA. 2016;316:191.
6. Manabe YC, Campbell JD, Sydnor E, et al. Immune reconstitution inflammatory syndrome: risk factors and treatment implications. J Acquir Immune Defic Syndr. 2007;46:456.
7. Müller M, Wandel S, Colebunders R, et al. Immune reconstitution inflammatory syndrome in patients starting antiretroviral therapy for HIV infection: a systematic review and meta-analysis. Lancet Infect Dis. 2010;10:251.
8. Navas E, Martín-Dávila P, Moreno L, et al. Paradoxical reactions of tuberculosis in patients with the acquired immunodeficiency syndrome who are treated with highly active antiretroviral therapy. Arch Intern Med. 2002;162:97.
9. Nelson AM, Manabe YC, Lucas SB. Immune reconstitution inflammatory syndrome (IRIS): what pathologists should know. Semin Diagn Pathol. 2017;34:340.

10. Nicolls DJ, King M, Holland D, et al. Intracranial tuberculomas developing while on therapy for pulmonary tuberculosis. Lancet Infect Dis. 2005;5:795.
11. Sempowski GD, Haynes BF. Immune reconstitution in patients with HIV infection. Annu Rev Med. 2002;53:269.
12. Shelburne SA 3rd, Hamill RJ, Rodriguez-Barradas MC, et al. Immune reconstitution inflammatory syndrome: emergence of a unique syndrome during highly active antiretroviral therapy. Medicine (Baltimore). 2002;81:213.
13. Sungkanuparph S, Jongwutiwes U, Kiertiburanakul S. Timing of cryptococcal immune reconstitution inflammatory syndrome after antiretroviral therapy in patients with AIDS and cryptococcal meningitis. J Acquir Immune Defic Syndr. 2007;45:595.

Index

Page numbers followed by *f* refer to figure, *fc* refer to flowchart and *t* refer to table.

B

C

D

E

I

K

L

M

N

O

P